Functional Electromechanical Dynamometry

Applications for Health and Sports Performance

Edited by Ángela Rodríguez-Perea and Ignacio J. Chirosa Rios

Routledge
Taylor & Francis Group
NEW YORK AND LONDON

First published 2025
by Routledge
605 Third Avenue, New York, NY 10158

and by Routledge
4 Park Square, Milton Park, Abingdon, Oxon, OX14 4RN

Routledge is an imprint of the Taylor & Francis Group, an informa business

ISBN: 978-1-032-54498-4 (hbk)
ISBN: 978-1-032-54499-1 (pbk)
ISBN: 978-1-003-42518-2 (ebk)

DOI: 10.4324/9781003425182

Typeset in Times New Roman
by Apex CoVantage, LLC

Functional Electromechanical Dynamometry

Human strength testing has advanced as technology has evolved from evaluating strength in a general and unspecialized way through to more scientific methods being applied to help performance and prevent injury. *Functional Electromechanical Dynamometry: Applications for Health and Sports Performance* continues this evolution by developing and presenting applications in the assessment and training of strength in humans, broadening the scope of information available to physical therapists, coaches, and physical trainers specializing in strength training.

Many of the current testing and training protocols are empirically based, with their roots in clinical medicine. They have been developed based on what the technology of the time allowed. With the application of new technologies, functional electromechanical dynamometry (FEMD), inertial devices, and mobile apps have seen the introduction of new testing protocols that outline how to assess strength in performance and the importance of muscle quality in injury prevention and treatment. Knowing how FEMDs work allows coaches, researchers, and health personnel to improve diagnoses and treatments for athletes and non-athletes and be able to better measure the stresses of the tasks that occur in everyday life, whether in daily activities or sports performance.

This new research book is key reading for sports science students, researchers, and academics and of specific relevance to those in the strength and conditioning or physiology fields as well as to anyone who wants to assess and improve musculoskeletal strength and muscle quality in humans.

Ángela Rodríguez-Perea is Doctor in Biomedicine from the University of Granada, Spain, and she holds a bachelor's degree in physical activity and sports sciences, an MSc in physical activity and sports research, and an MSc in secondary education with a specialization in physical education. Her research specialty interests are strength assessment, low back pain, core strength training, sports performance, and handball. Currently, she is a professor of Physical Education and Sports at the University of León, Spain. She is a member of the Pleokinetic Research Network and the IDAFISAD CTS-642 research group at the University of Granada, Spain.

Ignacio J. Chirosa Rios is a tenured professor of physical education and sports at the University of Granada, Spain. His research focuses on the evaluation and development of muscular strength and functional electromechanical dynamometry. Ignacio has published over 110 peer-reviewed journal articles and 14 PhD theses and has contributed to several research projects, about strength training applied to different populations from elite athletes to the elderly, including two as the principal investigator. He is actively involved in technology transfer, with multiple patents related to sports performance assessment tools, including a platform for FEMD. Ignacio also plays a significant role in academic leadership, coordinating doctoral programs and official master's programs at the University of Granada. He has been instrumental in creating international dynamometry laboratories across various countries, enhancing global research collaboration.

Routledge Research in Strength and Conditioning

Routledge Research in Strength and Conditioning brings together and showcases important new work in the field of strength and conditioning and related disciplines, including physiology, applied sport science, kinesiology, coaching and athletic training. The series features cutting edge research, dynamic interventions into established subjects and innovative studies on emerging topics.

Books within this series include the work of established and emerging researchers and practitioners from around the world, and can be single or multi-authored, or edited collections.

Available in this series:

Velocity-Based Training
Prescribing and Assessing the Effects of Resistance Training
Amador Garcia Ramos

Functional Electromechanical Dynamometry
Applications for Health and Sports Performance
Edited by Ángela Rodríguez-Perea and Ignacio J. Chirosa Rios

For more information about this series, please visit: Routledge Research in Strength and Conditioning - Book Series - Routledge & CRC Press

Contents

Figures

Tables

About the Contributors

Luis Javier Chirosa Ríos is a tenured professor at the University of Granada, Spain, specializing in strength training and functional electromyographic dynamometry. He leads the CTS642 "IDAFISAD" research group and the International "PLEOKINETIC" Network involving over 15 universities and 90 researchers. With 16 research projects and 172 indexed publications, he has pioneered the dynamometric mapping of the human body. He has supervised over 30 doctoral theses and advised companies like Myoquality Solutions S.L. A former professional handball player, he also has over 30 years of experience as a handball coach for professional teams.

Pedro Delgado-Floody, PhD, is an assistant professor of sports sciences at the Universidad de La Frontera, Chile. He has more than 150 *JCR* publications and was a postdoctoral fellow at the University of Granada under the Next Generation Fund of the European Union (2022–2024).

Álvaro Huerta Ojeda is professor of pedagogy in physical education and holds a bachelor's degree in education from the University of Playa Ancha (Chile). He has a master's degree in sports training from the Universidad Mayor (Chile) and a PhD in physical activity and health from the University of Granada (Spain). He is currently a full professor and director of the Research Center in Health, Physical Activity, and Sports (ISAFYD) at Universidad de las Américas (Chile).

Daniel Jerez-Mayorga has a master's degree in physical conditioning and health from the University of La Frontera, Chile, and is a doctor of biomedicine from the University of Granada, Spain. He is professor of physical education and kinesiologist. Currently, Daniel is a researcher at the Faculty of Sports Sciences at the University of Granada. He is member of the Pleokinetic Research Network and the IDAFISAD CTS-642 research group at the University of Granada. He has authored more than 150 indexed publications in the field of rehabilitation and sports sciences.

Daniel Jiménez-Lupión is a predoctoral research fellow at the Faculty of Sports Sciences, University of Granada, where he is preparing to become a university lecturer while conducting his doctoral thesis "Muscle Quality in Older Adults" in the Biomedicine PhD program. He holds a bachelor's degree in physical activity and sports sciences and has earned an MSc in sports science research and an MSc in secondary education with a specialization in physical education, both from the University of Granada. He has experience as a strength coach, focusing on strength training for health improvement and body composition.

Darío Martínez-García currently works as a lecturer at the University of Granada. His research is focused on strength training for performance enhancement and rehabilitation. He has published 35 articles indexed in *JCR* journals and contributed significantly to several national projects in both Chile and Spain.

Preface

The field of sports science has always been at the forefront of innovation, where the pursuit of human excellence meets the cutting edge of technology. This book represents a culmination of our shared commitment to exploring how technological advancements can revolutionize the way we understand and enhance athletic performance. Over the past week, we have worked tirelessly to distill our collective expertise and research into a coherent narrative that we hope will contribute meaningfully to the field.

Our focus in this book is on the integration of functional electromechanical dynamometers—a technology that, we believe, holds the potential to transform sports science. These devices, which precisely measure and analyze muscle performance, offer unprecedented insights into the biomechanics of movement, injury prevention, and rehabilitation. Throughout our careers, we have witnessed firsthand the limitations of traditional methods in assessing and improving athletic performance. This experience has driven us to explore how emerging technologies, particularly electromechanical dynamometry, and can overcome these limitations and open new frontiers in sports science.

This book is not merely a technical manual or a compilation of research findings. It is a dialogue between two passionate scientists who are eager to share the possibilities that this technology brings to the field. We aim to provide a comprehensive overview of the principles behind electromechanical dynamometry, its applications in various sports contexts, and the future directions we envision for this technology.

As coauthors, our collaboration has been built on a shared vision: to bridge the gap between theory and practice, and to offer practitioners, researchers, and students a resource that is both scientifically rigorous and practically relevant. Our discussions have been rich with ideas, challenges, and mutual respect, and this book is a testament to the synergy that can emerge from such collaboration.

We also recognize that the integration of new technology into established practices often comes with challenges. We have endeavored to address these head-on, offering insights into how functional electromechanical dynamometers can be implemented effectively in various settings, from elite sports training facilities to clinical environments. Our goal is to empower readers with the knowledge and tools to harness this technology for the benefit of athletes and the broader field of sports science.

We are deeply grateful to the many individuals who have supported us in this endeavor. From colleagues who provided invaluable feedback to the athletes and practitioners who allowed us to test and refine our ideas in real-world settings, this book is the result of collective effort. Their contributions have been instrumental in shaping the content and direction of this work.

As you read this book, we invite you to join us in exploring the exciting possibilities that functional electromechanical dynamometers bring to sports science. Whether you are a researcher, a coach, a physiotherapist, or a student, we hope that you will find value in the insights and innovations we have presented.

Thank you for embarking on this journey with us.

Sincerely,

Ángela Rodríguez-Perea and Ignacio J. Chirosa Rios

Section 1

Fundamentals of Strength Training

1 Introduction to Muscle Strength and Force in Sports Science

Ignacio J. Chirosa Rios

Introduction

In sports science, a deep and precise understanding of strength and force stands as the foundation for elevating athletic performance and prolonging sports careers. The meticulous application of these fundamental principles through ongoing research and evolving technology enables us to refine training regimens, enhance performance, and mitigate the risk of injuries more effectively than ever. By continuously pushing the envelope in understanding and application of these concepts, athletes can be equipped with the tools they need to exceed traditional performance limits and achieve new heights in their respective fields.

For decades, traditional tools such as free weights, resistance machines, and bodyweight exercises have been the cornerstone of strength training and rehabilitation. Free weights like barbells and dumbbells offer versatility and are fundamental for developing functional strength, allowing for natural movement patterns that engage stabilizing muscles (Kraemer & Ratamess, 2004). Resistance machines, on the other hand, provide a controlled environment where specific muscle groups can be isolated and trained with greater safety, particularly useful for beginners or during rehabilitation (Haff & Triplett, 2016).

However, as sports science and rehabilitation techniques have evolved, there has been a growing need for more sophisticated tools that can address the limitations of traditional equipment, such as the lack of precise resistance adjustment and real-time feedback (Haff & Nimphius, 2012). In response to this need, the integration of advanced motorized devices has emerged over the past decade as a transformative tool for enhancing athletic performance and optimizing recovery processes. These cutting-edge technologies, exemplified by devices like the Myoquality M1, the 1080 Motion system, and Kineo, offer unprecedented precision in training and rehabilitation. They enable athletes and physical therapists to target specific physical attributes with a level of accuracy and efficiency that was previously unattainable, marking a significant leap forward in the field (Oranchuk et al., 2020).

DOI: 10.4324/9781003425182-2

This book explores the benefits of motorized devices in sports science, with a particular focus on how they are revolutionizing strength training, power development, injury prevention, and rehabilitation fields (Oranchuk et al., 2020). Through case studies and scientific evidence, this text examines how these technologies contribute to improved outcomes for athletes and provide physical therapists with sophisticated tools to aid in patient recovery (Bittmann et al., 2022). This comprehensive knowledge not only optimizes individual athletes' potential but also redefines the parameters of possible achievements in sports (Haff & Nimphius, 2012). As understanding and application of strength and force advances, new benchmarks for athletic excellence are set, opening new possibilities for future generations of athletes, coaches, and therapists. This emphasis on cutting-edge technology in sports science serves as a catalyst for innovation, driving a more informed, health-conscious approach to sports training, performance enhancement, and active physical therapy. Strength and force not only are about the capacity to perform better in the short term but also involve enhancing an athlete's resilience, thereby fostering longevity (Kraemer & Ratamess, 2004).

Muscular strength, defined as the ability to exert force against external resistance, is a foundation of sports science (Stone, 1993). The application of this strength varies widely depending on the demands and dynamics of a particular sport or event. For example, athletes in track and field or gymnastics primarily contend with their body weight against gravity. In contrast, sports such as team handball or judo require athletes not only to control their own mass but also to manage the mass of an opponent during physical confrontations (Suchomel et al., 2016).

In activities like basketball or other team sports, as well as in CrossFit or weightlifting, the challenge extends to manipulating external objects—whether propelling a ball with precision or lifting weights to maximum capacity. The common thread across these diverse applications is the fundamental principle of force exertion, which directly influences the motion of a body in space (Suchomel & Comfort, 2022). This principle is succinctly captured by Newton's second law of motion, known as the law of acceleration. It states that force (F) is the product of mass (m) and acceleration (a), expressed as $F = ma$. According to this law, the acceleration imparted to a given mass is directly proportional to the force exerted and occurs in the same direction as that force.

This direct proportionality and alignment mean that enhancing muscular strength is not just about increasing force output but also about improving the efficiency and effectiveness of movement. Enhanced muscular strength allows athletes to generate greater acceleration with less effort, improving performance in dynamic activities such as sprinting or changing directions, and providing the sustained power needed for endurance-based activities. It also facilitates more precise and controlled movements, crucial in sports requiring high levels of skill and coordination, such as archery or golf.

Increasing muscular strength is also foundational to achieving optimal biomechanical leverage, which can significantly influence an athlete's ability to perform movements effectively. Strong muscles enhance an athlete's capacity to apply force advantageously, improving overall mechanical efficiency and performance outcomes (Steele et al., 2020a).

Muscular strength, therefore, is not just a singular trait but a dynamic capability that intersects various aspects of physical performance, from raw power and speed to technical precision and strategic execution (Kamarudin et al., 2022a). It underpins success in virtually every sport and is a primary focus of athletic training programs aiming to optimize athletes' physical potential across different sporting disciplines.

Advances in sports technology and research methodologies now allow sports scientists and trainers to analyze these mechanics more accurately than ever before. This ongoing evolution enables the development of training regimens finely tuned to individual athletes' needs, based on real-time data and biomechanical analysis. By applying these tailored training strategies, athletes can reach peak performance levels while minimizing injury risks, which often result from inadequate or misaligned training practices (Gabbett, 2016). Moreover, integrating motorized devices or functional electromechanical technology and research into the training process helps continuously monitor an athlete's performance and physiological responses. Tools such as functional dynamometers, force plates, and muscle electro-activity sensors provide immediate feedback that can be used to make instant adjustments to training methods. This level of detail ensures that every aspect of an athlete's training regimen is optimized for efficiency, effectiveness, and safety (Lambert & Borresen, 2010).

Expanding knowledge of strength and force allows sports professionals to push the boundaries of human performance. Each new discovery or technological breakthrough provides insights leading to unique training techniques, better performance-enhancing strategies, and innovative ways to prevent injuries. As this body of knowledge grows, it not only elevates individual athletes' performance but also raises the overall standards in sports disciplines and science. This applies not only to elite athletes but also to recreational sports enthusiasts, who can apply these scientifically backed principles to improve their performance and enjoyment of sports.

This comprehensive understanding and application of strength and force are not merely academic pursuits. They have real-world implications that can transform the landscape of sports training and performance. By pushing the boundaries of current sports performance, we pave the way for future generations of athletes and coaches to achieve new records and redefine what is possible in sports. Ultimately, the pursuit of knowledge in sports science serves as a catalyst for innovation across the entire spectrum of physical education and athletic competition, promoting a healthier, more scientifically engaged approach to sports training and performance enhancement (Bishop, 2008).

Beyond athletic performance, muscular strength and force play crucial roles in overall health and quality of life. Strong muscles are essential for maintaining mobility, supporting metabolic health, and enhancing daily functional capacity, which are critical for preventing chronic diseases and promoting longevity (Steele et al., 2020b). Enhanced muscular strength contributes to better metabolic health by improving glucose metabolism and insulin sensitivity, which are vital in preventing and managing conditions like type 2 diabetes (García-Hermoso et al., 2018). Additionally, maintaining muscle mass and strength is crucial for older adults to prevent sarcopenia, a condition characterized by loss of muscle mass and function, which can lead to frailty and increased risk of falls and fractures (Artero et al., 2011). Regular strength training can also enhance mental health by reducing symptoms of anxiety and depression, improving self-esteem, and enhancing cognitive function (Kamarudin et al., 2022b). These benefits underscore the importance of incorporating strength training into regular fitness routines for all age groups, not just athletes.

Understanding Strength and Force in Sports Science

In sports science, the concepts of "strength" and "force" are foundational and multifaceted, forming the foundation upon which much of athletic training and performance optimization is built. While these terms are frequently used interchangeably in everyday conversation, in the context of sports, they carry specific and distinct meanings that relate to physiological and biomechanical properties essential for athletic success.

"Strength" typically refers to the ability of muscle tissue to generate force against physical resistance, whether through lifting weights (free-weights or motorized resistance), resisting the force of gravity, or overcoming the inertia of stationary objects. It is a broad term that encompasses various types of strength, such as maximal strength, explosive strength, and endurance strength, each pertinent to different sports and activities. Maximal strength is the greatest force that muscles can exert in a single effort, explosive strength relates to the ability to exert maximal force in minimal time, and endurance strength is the ability to sustain repeated muscular actions or a single muscular action for extended periods (Cleather, 2021).

On the other hand, "force" is a more straightforward concept defined by physics as any interaction that, when unopposed, changes the motion of an object. In athletic contexts, this is exemplified as the power behind a sprinter's burst from the starting blocks or the impact of a gymnast's dismount. Understanding how to measure, manipulate, and maximize force is crucial for enhancing an athlete's performance and is closely tied to the laws of motion. In biomechanics, force is what causes an object—in this case, part of or the whole body—to accelerate or decelerate. It can be expressed through the basic equation $F = ma$ where F is the force applied, m is the mass of the object, and a is the acceleration.

A comprehensive understanding of strength requires a deeper knowledge of the force-velocity curve, which illustrates the inverse relationship between the force a muscle can generate and the velocity at which the external resistance or our body segments move and displace. This relationship is crucial for understanding how external resistance influences various aspects of strength. There are five distinct dimensions:

I. Maximal Strength: Maximal strength is represented at the high-force, low-velocity end of the force-velocity curve. Here, external resistance is typically very high, such as in heavy weightlifting exercises like squats, deadlifts, or bench presses. Because the load being manipulated is substantial, the velocity of movement is inherently slow. The relationship between external resistance and velocity is direct; as the resistance increases, the velocity of the bar decreases, but the force exerted by the muscles reaches its peak. Training for maximal strength involves lifting heavy loads at low speeds, focusing on maximizing force output against significant external resistance.

II. Maximum Power: Power occupies the middle of the force-velocity curve, where there is an optimal balance between force and velocity. Some authors call this dimension strength-speed (Suchomel & Comfort, 2022). At this point, external resistance is moderate, allowing the athlete to move at a faster pace while still generating substantial force. Power is crucial for explosive movements such as jumping, sprinting, or Olympic lifts, where both force and velocity are essential. The external resistance is enough to require significant effort but not so high as to slow down the movement excessively. Training for power typically involves exercises that optimize the relationship between force and velocity, such as plyometrics, ballistic movements, and Olympic lifts, where the goal is to produce the highest possible force at relatively high velocities.

III. Speed-Strength: Speed-strength lies at the low-force, high-velocity end of the force-velocity curve. Here, the external resistance is low, allowing for maximum movement speed. This dimension of strength is important for activities that require rapid muscle contractions with minimal load, such as sprinting or agility drills. As external resistance decreases, the velocity of movement increases, and the focus shifts to generating force quickly rather than producing maximum force. Training for speed strength involves exercises that emphasize rapid, high-velocity movements, often with little to no external resistance, to improve the speed of muscular contractions.

IV. Strength Endurance: Strength endurance is somewhat independent of the force-velocity extremes but is crucial for sustaining muscle contractions over time against moderate external resistance. In activities like rowing, cycling, or distance running, the external resistance is typically consistent and moderate, requiring the athlete to maintain a steady force output over an extended period. While not directly tied to the peak force or velocity, strength endurance training focuses on the ability to resist fatigue and maintain force production over time, often involving higher repetitions with moderate resistance.

V. Endurance of Strength: More than just a dimension, endurance of strength is a critical capacity that must be developed across all expressions of force. While it is often discussed as a separate aspect of strength, endurance of strength underpins the ability to sustain force production over time, whether in maximal strength efforts, power-based movements, or activities requiring speed-strength.

Endurance of strength is essential because it ensures that an athlete can maintain their performance across prolonged periods or repeated efforts. For example, in maximal strength, endurance allows an athlete to sustain high levels of force output during multiple sets of heavy lifting. In power-based activities, it enables the athlete to continue generating explosive movements without a significant drop in performance as fatigue sets in. In speed strength, endurance helps maintain rapid force production across repeated sprints or agility drills.

Developing endurance of strength requires integrating various training methods that challenge the muscles to resist fatigue while maintaining force output. This might involve higher repetitions with moderate weights, circuit training, or specific endurance drills tailored to the demands of the sport. By cultivating this capacity across all forms of strength, athletes can improve their ability to perform consistently at high levels, regardless of the duration or intensity of the activity. In essence, endurance of strength is the foundation that supports all other dimensions of strength, ensuring that force production can be sustained and effective in real-world athletic scenarios. It is a crucial aspect of comprehensive strength training that contributes significantly to overall athletic performance and resilience.

Moreover, understanding the relationship between the force-velocity curve and external resistance allows athletes and coaches to design training programs that specifically target different points on the curve. By manipulating external resistance—whether increasing it to enhance maximal strength or reducing it to focus on speed strength—training can be tailored to meet the specific demands of the sport. For instance, athletes aiming to improve their power must find the optimal balance between force and velocity by adjusting external resistance to a level that allows for both substantial force production and rapid movement. Conversely, those focusing on maximal strength will work with heavier loads to push the limits of force production at lower velocities.

Thus, the force-velocity curve is the essential metric in strength and conditioning and sports science, highlighting the relationship between the force a muscle generates and the velocity of its contractions. By examining the key dimensions—maximal strength, maximum power, speed-strength, and strength endurance (also consider the capacity of each dimension, endurance of strength)—athletes and trainers can unlock a wide array of strategies to enhance various expressions of force. Integrated training programs that address all these dimensions—through heavy resistance training, plyometric exercises, and high-repetition workouts—ensure balanced development and optimal performance tailored to the specific demands of any sport or physical activity.

Physiological Basis of Strength and Force

While this book doesn't delve deeply into the physiological basis of strength and force, it provides a concise overview of the factors that influence force production and its subsequent development. Force production and the different expressions of strength are complex processes primarily influenced by the muscular, neurological, skeletal, and fascial systems of the body. Each system plays a critical role in the mechanics of movement and performance:

a) Muscular System: The muscle fibers, categorized into type I slow-twitch and type II fast-twitch, respond uniquely under various types of strength training. Type II fibers are especially crucial for generating the high levels of force required in explosive movements, such as sprinting or jumping, due to their rapid contraction capabilities.
b) Neurological System: The nervous system is essential for effective force production and strength expression. It regulates the recruitment of motor units, which are groups of muscle fibers controlled by a single motor neuron. This system is also responsible for the precise coordination of muscle actions, allowing for complex movements required in sports and other physical activities.
c) Skeletal System: The bones provide the necessary leverage for force exertion and play a pivotal role in the transmission of forces generated by muscular contractions. The arrangement of bones and joints determines the mechanical advantage with which forces can be applied, impacting everything from lifting heavy weights to striking a ball.
d) Fascial System: The fascia, a dense connective tissue network that envelops and interconnects muscles, bones, and organs, also plays a vital role in force transmission. It acts as a mediator that transmits the mechanical load throughout the body, contributing to the overall structural integrity and coordinated movement. The fascia's ability to store and release elastic potential energy is especially important in movements that require the stretching and shortening of muscles, enhancing both the efficiency and effectiveness of force application. This connective tissue's properties are crucial for maintaining posture and providing the necessary tensional network through which muscles can exert force more effectively.

Biomechanical Principles

Understanding the biomechanical principles that govern movement and force application is essential for optimizing athletic performance and other areas of sports science. Incorporating insights from the microstructures like muscle fibers to the macrostructures of muscle chains and joint mechanics allows for a comprehensive approach to enhancing physical capabilities. A rundown of these principles follows, beginning with the microstructural elements:

Biomechanics of Muscle Fibers

Muscle fibers, the fundamental units of muscle, contain myofibrils made up of contractile proteins—actin and myosin. During muscle contractions, these proteins interact in a process fueled by ATP energy, sliding past each other to shorten the muscle. The entire muscle fiber is wrapped in fascia, which transmits the generated force to the bones, facilitating body movements (Lieber & Friden, 2000). The capacity of muscle fibers to generate force is significantly influenced by their cross-sectional area. Type II fast-twitch fibers, known for their larger size and rapid contraction capabilities, are especially adept at producing force. This can be enhanced through strength training that induces muscular hypertrophy and increases contractile efficiency (Staron et al., 1988). Studies have shown that resistance training significantly increases the size and strength of fast-twitch fibers, thereby improving overall muscle force production (Schoenfeld, 2010).

Lastly, efficient force production is heavily dependent on neuromuscular coordination. Through training, the synchronization of muscle contractions and the firing rates of motor neurons can be enhanced, resulting in more powerful and coordinated movements across multiple muscle groups. Research indicates that specific strength and power training can enhance motor unit recruitment and firing frequency, contributing to improved athletic performance (Gabriel et al., 2006).

Biomechanical Principles Applied to Force Production

a) Leverage: This principle uses the arrangement of bones and joints as levers to maximize force output and minimize the risk of injury. By manipulating the length and position of the lever arm, athletes can achieve greater mechanical advantage, crucial in sports that involve lifting or throwing. The biomechanics of leverage in sports have been extensively studied, showing that optimal lever arm length can significantly enhance performance (Komi, 2003).
b) Torque: Torque is the rotational force applied by the muscles around a joint. It plays a critical role in any sport requiring turning movements, such as golf or tennis. The torque generated by muscle contractions can be enhanced

by increasing the force applied or by extending the distance from the joint at which force is applied (Zatsiorsky & Kraemer, 2006). Targeted training can improve torque production, as demonstrated in various studies, thus enhancing performance in rotational sports (Elliott et al., 1999).

c) Elasticity: Muscle tissues exhibit elasticity, allowing them to store and release energy efficiently. This elastic property is fundamental in explosive movements like jumps or sprints, where the rapid shortening of elongated muscle tissues converts potential energy into kinetic energy, propelling the athlete forward (Kubo et al., 2000). Research has shown that plyometric training can significantly enhance the elastic properties of muscles, contributing to improved explosive performance (Markovic, 2007).

Macrostructures and Muscle Chains

The interaction between individual muscles and the broader network of muscle chains underscores the complexity of human biomechanics. Muscle chains refer to groups of muscles that work together to produce movement in a coordinated and efficient manner. Training that focuses on entire muscle chains rather than isolated muscles can lead to more functional strength and dynamic stability, which are essential for high-level performance and injury prevention (Myers, 2001). Studies support that integrated training approaches enhance overall athletic performance by improving the synergy and functionality of muscle chains (Kibler et al., 2006).

Principles of Sports Training

The application of strength and force in sports training is governed by several key principles that ensure athletes develop the right type of strength for their sports and progressively enhance their capacity in a structured manner. These principles not only help in achieving peak physical performance but also play a crucial role in injury prevention.

Specificity

Training adaptations are specific to the stimuli applied, which means that training should closely mimic the movements, energy systems, and demands of the sport. For example, a sprinter should focus on explosive leg exercises that simulate the actions of sprinting to enhance power and speed.

Overload

To improve strength and endurance, the body must be challenged by a workload greater than what it's accustomed to. This can be achieved by increasing the resistance, the number of repetitions, or the intensity of the exercises. Overload should be applied progressively to stimulate continuous adaptation without causing injury or excessive fatigue.

Progression

The intensity or volume of training should gradually increase over time to continue challenging the body and prevent plateaus in performance improvement. Progression can be managed through careful monitoring of performance metrics and adjusting the training load accordingly.

Individualization

Each athlete has unique physical capabilities, recovery needs, and responses to training stimuli. Strength training programs should be customized to meet the individual needs of athletes, considering factors such as age, gender, fitness level, and sport-specific goals.

Reversibility

Reversibility refers to the loss of fitness that occurs after a period of reduced or no physical activity. It underscores the "use it or lose it" nature of fitness attributes like muscle strength, endurance, and flexibility. In the context of strength training, maintaining a consistent training regimen is critical because the gains in muscle strength and neuromuscular coordination can regress if training is not sustained.

Important Concepts in Muscle Strength and Force Production

Comprehension of muscle strength and force production is fundamental in sports science, physical therapy, and general fitness. Several key concepts are crucial to comprehend how muscles generate force and how this force translates into movement and strength. Here are the most important concepts:

1. Motor Unit Recruitment. A motor unit comprises an alpha motor neuron and all the muscle fibers it controls. The force's magnitude and rate are directly linked to the number and type of motor units activated. According to the classic study of Henneman et al. (1965), motor units are recruited sequentially from smallest to largest based on the demands of the activity. For instance, low-force demands initially engage smaller, slow-twitch Type I muscle fibers. If the activity requires greater force and a faster rate

of force development (RFD), larger, fast-twitch Type IIa and IIx fibers are subsequently recruited. This recruitment pattern is consistent across different types of muscle actions, including slow, graded, isometric, and ballistic movements. However, during rapid, ballistic movements, the thresholds for motor unit recruitment are often lower due to the increased demand for rapid force development, suggesting that training that includes high-velocity movements can be particularly effective for improving muscle strength, RFD, and overall power.

2. Rate Coding. The firing frequency, or the rate at which neural impulses are sent from the α-motor neuron to the muscle fibers, can significantly modify force production properties following motor unit recruitment. Research indicates that increasing the firing frequency can boost force production by as much as 300%–1,500% (Enoka, 1995). Furthermore, higher initial firing rates are associated with an increase in doublet discharges, which can significantly influence RFD. Training modalities that enhance the firing frequency, such as ballistic exercises, have been shown to significantly improve neuromuscular efficiency within just 12 weeks (Van Cutsem et al., 1998).
3. Motor Unit Synchronization. Motor unit synchronization, the simultaneous activation of multiple motor units, can enhance force production. While its role is more closely related to RFD than to force magnitude, studies have shown that strength training can increase motor unit synchronization, potentially aiding in rapid muscle actions (Semmler, 2002; Semmler et al., 2000). Notably, tasks that require dynamic movement tend to show improved synchronization, particularly after heavy strength training.
4. Neuromuscular Inhibition. Neuromuscular inhibition refers to the reduction in voluntary neural drive to muscle groups during actions and can impede force production. This phenomenon is often influenced by neural feedback from muscle and joint receptors. However, studies suggest that heavy strength training can reduce this inhibition by down-regulating Ib afferent feedback to the spinal motor neuron pool, thereby enhancing force production (Aagaard et al., 2000). Further research indicates that such training also increases neural drive from both spinal and supraspinal levels, decreasing neuromuscular inhibition and enhancing RFD (Aagaard et al., 2002).
5. Muscle Fiber Types. Muscle fibers are categorized into two main types:

    - Type I (Slow-Twitch): These fibers are more fatigue-resistant and are primarily used during endurance activities. They generate less force but can sustain activity for longer durations.
    - Type II (Fast-Twitch): These fibers are larger, generate more force, and fatigue more quickly. They are important for short, explosive movements like sprinting or jumping. Type II fibers are further divided into Type IIa and Type IIx, with varying capabilities for speed and endurance.

6. Length-Tension Relationship. The force a muscle can produce is also affected by its length during contraction. There is an optimal muscle length at which the force production is maximal, determined by the maximum overlap of actin and myosin filaments within the muscle cells. Deviations from this length can reduce the efficiency of force production.
7. Force-Velocity Relationship. The force-velocity relationship describes how the velocity at which a muscle fiber shortens impacts the force it can produce. Generally, the faster a muscle fiber shortens, the lower the force it can produce, and vice versa. This relationship is crucial for designing training regimens tailored to specific athletic needs or rehabilitation goals.
8. Eccentric, Concentric, and Isometric Contractions. Muscle contractions are categorized based on the movement of the muscle:
   - Concentric Contractions: Muscle shortening while producing force—typical in lifting a weight.
   - Eccentric Contractions: Muscle lengthens while producing force—important for controlled lowering of weights.
   - Isometric Contractions: Muscle generates force without changing length—seen when holding a static position.
9. Biomechanical and Structural Factors. Biomechanical aspects such as joint angles, body posture, and the mechanical advantage offered by different parts of the skeletal system play significant roles in how effectively force is produced and applied during various movements.

How to Improve Strength and Force Production

While upcoming chapters will explore this topic more deeply, to effectively improve strength and force production capabilities, a multifaceted approach is necessary, incorporating structured training regimens, well-planned programs, sufficient recovery periods, and focused psychological conditioning. This comprehensive strategy ensures that all aspects of health and performance are addressed.

Structured Strength Training

To continually challenge the muscles and stimulate growth, gradual increases in weight, frequency, or the number of repetitions in a training routine are necessary. Additionally, a variety of exercises that target different muscle groups promote balanced strength development. These include free weights, machines, resistance bands, bodyweight exercises, pneumatic resistance, and motorized resistance. Using periodization—implementing a training schedule that varies in intensity, volume, and types of exercises over different periods—optimizes gains and prevents plateaus. Periodization typically involves cycles of hypertrophy, strength, power, and endurance phases.

Optimal Technique and Biomechanics

Learning and maintaining correct technique is crucial for maximizing force output and minimizing injury risk. This is complemented by understanding the impact of correct body position and learning to manipulate angles can significantly enhance the effectiveness of force production.

Muscle Fiber Recruitment

Compound movements include exercises like squats, deadlifts, and bench presses that engage multiple muscle groups. These movements help improve neuromuscular coordination and increase overall strength. Explosive training such as plyometrics and Olympic lifts (like snatch and clean and jerk) are effective for developing power and velocity by enhancing fast-twitch muscle fiber recruitment.

Adequate Recovery

Adequate rest between training sessions and sufficient sleep are vital for muscle recovery and growth. The target should be seven to nine hours of quality sleep per night. Active recovery—light activity and mobility work—should take place on rest days to promote circulation and muscle healing.

Psychological Factors

Developing resilience and mental strategies to handle the physical demands of training and competition is another essential component of training. Techniques like visualization, goal setting, and stress management can help athletes reach their maximum potential. Consistency and motivation play a large role in building strength and power since this is a long-term process that requires consistent effort and dedication. Setting short-term goals can help maintain motivation over time.

Monitoring and Adjusting

Regularly assessing strength gains through performance metrics (like max lifts) and physiological tests determines the effectiveness of a training regimen. Adjusting training programs based on progress, plateaus, and physical feedback is necessary. Listening to one's body and adapting training and recovery strategies accordingly is crucial for continued improvement.

Measurement and Evaluation

Understanding the primary methods used to measure and evaluate strength and force production is essential for effectively assessing an athlete's performance capabilities and designing appropriate training programs to enhance these critical attributes. Each method offers unique insights into different aspects of strength and force, enabling a comprehensive evaluation of an athlete's physical condition and progress. An overview of the primary methods used to measure and evaluate strength and force production follows.

Maximal Strength Tests

- One-Repetition Maximum (1RM): This is the most common test for measuring maximal strength, especially in resistance training. It determines the maximum load an individual can lift for one complete repetition of a given exercise, such as a bench press or squat.
- 1RM in the Concentric Phase: The concentric phase of the 1RM test involves the muscle shortening as it contracts to lift the weight. For example, in a bench press, the concentric phase occurs as the lifter pushes the barbell away from their chest, extending their arms. This phase is critical for assessing the ability to generate force to overcome resistance and move it. The maximal weight lifted during this phase is indicative of the lifter's maximal concentric strength.
- 1RM in the Eccentric Phase: The eccentric phase of the 1RM test involves the muscle lengthening while still under tension, as it controls the lowering of the weight. In the bench press, this phase occurs as the lifter lowers the barbell back down to their chest. The eccentric phase tests the ability to resist and control the weight, which often involves greater force production compared to the concentric phase. Maximal strength in this phase is essential for preventing injuries and enhancing overall muscle development.
- Isometric Strength Testing: Isometric strength testing measures the maximum force exerted without movement, often using a dynamometer. This test is particularly useful for assessing strength in populations where movement may pose a risk or where specific joint angles need evaluation. Unlike dynamic tests like the 1RM, isometric tests focus on the force produced at a specific joint angle, providing valuable information about muscle strength and function in that particular position.

Concepts of Pushing and Holding

In the context of maximal strength tests, understanding the concepts of pushing and holding is essential for a comprehensive evaluation:

- Pushing

  Pushing refers to the dynamic action of exerting force to move an object or resistance, which is exemplified by the 1RM test. This test involves both the concentric and eccentric phases of a lift, requiring the individual to generate maximal force to overcome and control resistance. The ability to push maximally is indicative of the person's dynamic strength and capacity to perform tasks involving movement against resistance.

- Holding
  Holding, on the other hand, involves maintaining a static position against resistance, as seen in isometric strength testing. This test measures the ability to exert maximal force without changing the muscle length or joint angle. Holding is crucial for evaluating static strength, which is important for activities requiring stability and endurance in specific positions. This form of strength is particularly relevant in rehabilitation settings, where movement might be contraindicated, and in sports or tasks that require sustained muscle contractions.

Isokinetic Testing

These tests utilize specialized machines (isokinetic dynamometers) that measure the force and torque an individual can produce at a constant speed. This method is highly precise and allows for detailed analysis of muscle function and strength across a range of motion, making it invaluable in rehabilitation settings.

Functional Movement Tests

Functional movement tests assess strength through functional movements, which can provide more sport-specific insights. Examples include:

- Vertical Jump Test: Measures lower body explosive strength.
- Medicine Ball Throw: Tests upper body strength and power.
- Pull-Up or Push-Up Tests: Evaluate muscular endurance and upper body strength.

Force Plates

These advanced devices measure the forces generated by a body standing on or moving across them. Force plates can provide detailed data on ground reaction forces, the timing of movements, and balance, which are essential for high-performance sports and biomechanical analysis.

Electromyography

Electromyography (EMG) measures the electrical activity produced by muscles during contraction. It provides insights into which muscles are being activated during different exercises and the intensity of muscle engagement, offering valuable data for optimizing athletic training and rehabilitation.

Handheld Dynamometers

These portable devices are used to measure the force output of different muscle groups. They are particularly useful in clinical settings for assessing muscle strength and recovery following an injury.

Field Tests

Field tests are simple tests that can be conducted without specialized equipment. Examples include the timed sit-up test for core strength, the handgrip strength test using a handgrip dynamometer, and various plyometric tests.

Technological Integration

Current technology such as wearable sensors and mobile apps are increasingly used to provide real-time, actionable data on an athlete's performance during training or competition. These tools can track movement efficiency, force application, and overall physical output.

Psychological Assessment

While they don't directly measure physical strength or force, psychological assessments can evaluate an athlete's mental toughness and readiness, which significantly influence performance in strength and power sports.

Longitudinal Tracking

Monitoring changes over time through repeated testing is crucial for assessing the effectiveness of training programs and making necessary adjustments based on objective data.

Strength and Force Production Challenges and Considerations Throughout a Lifespan

Strength and force production undergo significant changes throughout a person's life and each phase presents unique challenges requiring specialized training, rehabilitation, and everyday life management. Recognizing these shifts is essential for tailoring approaches that effectively support an individual's health and physical capabilities at every age. A summary of key points regarding the challenges and considerations of maintaining and improving strength and force production through different stages of life follows:

1. Childhood and Adolescence
   During childhood and adolescence, growth occurs rapidly, and strength training should be carefully managed to avoid injuries to growth plates.

In early childhood, the development of motor skills is the priority. Later, the focus of training should be on proper technique rather than the development of strength through lifting heavy weights. Progressive resistance exercises can be introduced as children mature. The psychological component of exercise at these ages is important. Maintaining a fun and engaging environment is crucial to fostering a lifelong interest in physical activity.

2. Early Adulthood
During early adulthood, people typically reach peak muscle mass and strength. Training can be intensified, with a focus on maximizing strength and power through structured resistance training programs. However, balancing training with other responsibilities like career and family can be challenging. For amateur athletes efficient, high-intensity functional training can be effective during this stage of life.
3. Middle Age
As people enter their 30s and 40s, maintaining muscle mass and strength becomes a challenge due to natural physiological changes. Resistance training is especially important to counteract the natural decline in muscle strength and metabolic rate. Additionally, issues such as joint health and the onset of chronic conditions (like arthritis or cardiovascular disease) may require modifications to training routines.
4. Older Adults
Older adults have different concerns yet again when it comes to changes in strength and force production. Aging is associated with a progressive loss of muscle mass and strength, known as sarcopenia, leading to increased frailty and a higher risk of falls. Therefore, a key focus of strength training for seniors should focus on maintaining mobility, balance, and functional independence. Exercises often emphasize lower-intensity, high-repetition workouts that improve stability and endurance. Finally, older adults may need more time for recovery between sessions, and exercises may need to be modified to accommodate physical limitations or medical conditions.
5. Special Considerations Across All Ages
Independent of one's age, genetic factors, lifestyle choices, and pre-existing health conditions significantly influence strength capabilities and training effectiveness. Personalized training programs are essential. Adequate nutrition at every age mustn't be overlooked, including sufficient protein intake and essential nutrients, which are crucial for muscle repair and growth at any age.

Regardless of age group, proper form and technique are vital to avoid injuries. When injuries occur, rehabilitation and recovery protocols should be adjusted according to age and health status.

Finally, regular assessments track the progress and effectiveness of strength training programs, and adjustments should be made as needed based on age-related changes and individual responses.

Effective application of strength and force in sports training comes with its challenges. Balancing the need for intense training to maximize force and strength with the risk of overtraining and injury is critical in both professional and amateur athletes, and those wishing to live long, healthy lives.

The following chapters of this book explore all the concepts in greater detail, providing evidence, case studies, and best practices for achieving strength and force production for specialists from many disciplines.

References

Aagaard, P., Simonsen, E. B., Andersen, J. L., Magnusson, S. P., Bojsen-Møller, F., & Dyhre-Poulsen, P. (2000). Antagonist muscle coactivation during isokinetic knee extension. *Scandinavian Journal of Medicine & Science in Sports*, *10*(2), 58–67. https://doi.org/10.1034/j.1600-0838.2000.010002058.x

Aagaard, P., Simonsen, E. B., Andersen, J. L., Magnusson, S. P., & Dyhre-Poulsen, P. (2002). Increased rate of force development and neural drive of human skeletal muscle following resistance training. *Journal of Applied Physiology*, *93*(4), 1318–1326. https://doi.org/10.1152/japplphysiol.00283.2002

Artero, E. G., et al. (2011). A prospective study of muscular strength and all-cause mortality in men with hypertension. *Journal of the American College of Cardiology*, *57*(18), 1831–1837. https://doi.org/10.1016/j.jacc.2010.12.025

Bishop, D. (2008). An applied research model for the sport sciences. *Sports Medicine*, *38*(3), 253–263.

Bittmann, F., Schaefer, L., & Rudroff, T. (2022). Adaptive force: A potential new method for detecting deficits in neuromuscular performance. *Frontiers in Physiology*, *13*, 821619. https://doi.org/10.3389/fphys.2022.821619

Cleather, D. (2021). *Force: The Biomechanics of Training*. Chequia: Independently Published.

Elliott, B., et al. (1999). The biomechanical principles applied to human movement. *Australian Journal of Science and Medicine in Sport*, *27*(4), 47–53.

Enoka, R. M. (1995). Morphological features and activation patterns of motor units. *Journal of Clinical Neurophysiology*, *12*(4), 538–559. https://doi.org/10.1097/00004691-199507000-00009

Gabbett, T. J. (2016). The training—injury prevention paradox: Should athletes be training smarter and harder? *British Journal of Sports Medicine, 50*, 273–280.

Gabriel, D. A., Kamen, G., & Frost, G. (2006). Neural adaptations to resistive exercise: Mechanisms and recommendations for training practices. *Sports Medicine*, *36*(2), 133–149.

García-Hermoso, A., Ramírez-Vélez, R., & Izquierdo, M. (2018). Is muscular fitness associated with future health benefits in children and adolescents? A systematic review and meta-analysis of longitudinal studies. *Sports Medicine*, *49*, 1079–1094. https://doi.org/10.1007/s40279-018-01092-6

Haff, G. G., & Nimphius, S. (2012). Training principles for power. *Strength and Conditioning Journal*, *34*(6), 2–12. https://doi.org/10.1519/SSC.0b013e31826db3cf

Haff, G. G., & Triplett, N. T. (2016). *Essentials of Strength Training and Conditioning* (4th ed.). Human Kinetics.

Henneman, E., Somjen, G., & Carpenter, D. O. (1965). Functional significance of cell size in spinal motoneurons. *Journal of Neurophysiology*, *28*(3), 560–580. https://doi.org/10.1152/jn.1965.28.3.560

Kamarudin, N. A., Abdullah, M. R., Musa, R. M., Eswaramoorthi, V., Maliki, A., Ab Rasid, A. M., & Nadzmi, A. (2022a). Physical fitness performance comparison based on body mass index between individual sports and team sports athletes. *International Journal of Academic Research in Progressive Education and Development*, *11*(1), 342–359.

Kamarudin, S., Boo, N. Y., Nor Aripin, K. N., Nor Azman, K., & Cheang, S. K. (2022b). Effects of a structured physical exercise program on cognitive function, physical performance, and mental health among older adults: A randomized controlled trial. *Clinical Interventions in Aging*, *17*, 621–630. https://doi.org/10.2147/CIA.S355255

Kibler, W. B., et al. (2006). The role of the scapula in athletic shoulder function. *The American Journal of Sports Medicine*, *34*(3), 362–370.

Komi, P. V. (2003). *Strength and Power in Sport: Encyclopedia of Sports Medicine*. Blackwell Science.

Kraemer, W. J., & Ratamess, N. A. (2004). Fundamentals of resistance training: Progression and exercise prescription. *Medicine & Science in Sports & Exercise*, *36*(4), 674–688. https://doi.org/10.1249/01.MSS.0000121945.36635.61

Kubo, K., et al. (2000). Elastic properties of muscle-tendon complex in long-distance runners. *European Journal of Applied Physiology*, *81*(3), 181–187.

Lambert, M. I., & Borresen, J. (2010). Measuring training load in sports. *International Journal of Sports Physiology and Performance*, *5*(3), 406–411.

Lieber, R. L., & Friden, J. (2000). Functional and clinical significance of skeletal muscle architecture. *Muscle & Nerve*, *23*(11), 1647–1666.

Markovic, G. (2007). Does plyometric training improve vertical jump height? A meta-analytical review. *British Journal of Sports Medicine*, *41*(6), 349–355.

Myers, T. W. (2001). *Anatomy Trains: Myofascial Meridians for Manual and Movement Therapists*. Elsevier.

Oranchuk, D. J., Storey, A. G., Nelson, A. R., & Cronin, J. B. (2020). Isometric training and long-term adaptations: Effects of muscle length, intensity, and intent: A systematic review. *Scandinavian Journal of Medicine & Science in Sports*, *30*(5), 774–784. https://doi.org/10.1111/sms.13621

Schoenfeld, B. J. (2010). The mechanisms of muscle hypertrophy and their application to resistance training. *Journal of Strength and Conditioning Research*, *24*(10), 2857–2872.

Semmler, J. G. (2002). Motor unit synchronization and neuromuscular performance. *Exercise and Sport Sciences Reviews*, *30*(1), 8–14. https://doi.org/10.1097/00003677-200201000-00003

Semmler, J. G., Sale, M. V., Meyer, F. G., & Nordstrom, M. A. (2000). Motor unit coherence and its relation with synchrony are influenced by training. *Journal of Neurophysiology*, *84*(1), 462–471. https://doi.org/10.1152/jn.2000.84.1.462

Staron, R. S., et al. (1988). Muscle hypertrophy and fast fiber type conversions in heavy resistance-trained women. *European Journal of Applied Physiology and Occupational Physiology*, *57*(1), 71–77.

Steele, J., Fisher, J., & Crawford, D. (2020a). Does increasing an athletes' strength improve sports performance? A critical review with suggestions to help answer this, and other, causal questions in sport science. *Journal of Trainology*, *9*(1), 20–32.

Steele, J., Fisher, J., Skivington, M., Dunn, C., Arnold, J., Tew, G., Batterham, A. M., Nunan, D., O'Driscoll, J. M., Mann, S., Beedie, C., Jobson, S., Smith, D., Vigotsky, A., Phillips, S., Estabrooks, P., & Stokes, K. A. (2020b). A higher effort-based paradigm in physical activity and exercise for public health: Making the case for a greater emphasis on resistance training. *BMC Public Health*, *20*(1), 1–11. https://doi.org/10.1186/s12889-020-09452-z

Stone, M. H. (1993). Position statement: Explosive exercises and training. *National Strength and Conditioning Association Journal*, *15*, 7–15.

Suchomel, T. J., & Comfort, P. (2022). Developing muscular strength and power. In *Advanced Strength and Conditioning* (pp. 13–39). Routledge.

Suchomel, T. J., Nimphius, S., & Stone, M. H. (2016). The importance of muscular strength in athletic performance. *Sports Medicine*, *46*(10), 1419–1449.

Van Cutsem, M., Duchateau, J., & Hainaut, K. (1998). Changes in single motor unit behavior contribute to the increase in contraction speed after dynamic training in humans. *Journal of Physiology*, *513*(1), 295–305. https://doi.org/10.1111/j.1469-7793.1998.295by.x

Zatsiorsky, V. M., & Kraemer, W. J. (2006). *Science and Practice of Strength Training*. Human Kinetics.

2 Expressions of Force

Ignacio J. Chirosa Rios

Introduction

Strength is a multifaceted ability that is expressed in various ways both in sports and in daily life. In sports, strength adapts to the specific demands of each discipline, allowing athletes to maximize their performance. In everyday life, strength is essential for carrying out daily tasks efficiently and safely, contributing to functionality and quality of life. Understanding how strength manifests and can be improved in these contexts is crucial for designing effective training and rehabilitation programs tailored to individual needs.

The mechanics of strength is an intricate interplay between force, motion, and the human body's capabilities. It involves far more than just muscle contractions; it is a complicated system governed by the principles of physics and the complexity of human physiology (Siff & Verkhoshansky, 1999). Muscle architecture, including fiber type and the specific points of muscle attachment, plays a pivotal role in determining an individual's strength potential and force output (Lieber, 2010). For instance, longer muscle fibers have the capacity to generate greater force by contracting over a larger distance, while the angle at which muscles attach to bones influences the leverage and mechanical advantage each muscle can exert (Zatsiorsky & Prilutsky, 2012).

However, the expression of strength is not merely a function of muscle structure. The nervous system is integral to the development of strength, particularly through neural adaptations that enhance performance. In the early stages of strength training, improvements in force production often result from the nervous system's ability to recruit more motor units and synchronize their firing patterns, leading to significant gains in strength even before visible changes in muscle size occur (Enoka, 2008). This chapter delves deep into the intricate dynamics of force expression, not only exploring the well-established concepts of static and dynamic expressions of its variants but also introducing the nuanced categories of holding and pushing. By dissecting these fundamental concepts, this section sets the stage for a comprehensive understanding tailored for specialists in strength and conditioning as well as sports scientists and physical therapists.

DOI: 10.4324/9781003425182-3

At the heart of understanding force expressions in sports science lies a robust grasp of basic physics principles: force, work, energy, and power. These principles are the framework upon which all athletic movements and training regimens are built. Force, a vector quantity that initiates an object's movement or causes it to stop is the primary focus in sports biomechanics. This chapter explores how these forces—whether exerted by a sprinter on the track or a weightlifter during a lift—translate into work (force applied over distance) and how energy transformations are crucial for different sporting tasks. Additionally, the concept of power—the rate at which work is done—is dissected to highlight its importance in sports where time is a critical factor.

From Traditional Classification and Definitions of Force Expressions to a Modern, Integrated Approach

Force expressions refer to the various ways in which force is generated, exerted, and utilized by the human body in response to physical demands (Tous-Fajardo, 1999). These expressions are foundational to all movements, whether in sports, daily activities, or rehabilitation. Understanding force expressions is crucial for developing precise and effective training programs, enhancing athletic performance, and ensuring efficient recovery in rehabilitation settings.

Vittori (1990) classified the expression of force into two primary categories: Passive and Active. He further subdivided the Active category into distinct expressions, including Maximum Dynamic Force (MDF), Maximum Explosive Force (MEF), Specific Task Force, Explosive Reactive Force (ERF), and Explosive Reactive-Reflex Force (ERRF). Each of these subcategories encompasses specific characteristics and applications, providing a comprehensive framework for understanding the diverse demands of different sports. In the following analysis, each concept and its derivatives will be explored in detail to equip coaches and sports scientists with the knowledge needed to effectively address and optimize performance across various athletic disciplines.

Passive Force Expressions

Passive Force Expressions involve force production without movement, where muscles generate tension but do not change length. This type of force is crucial for stability, posture, and tasks that require holding positions against resistance.

Maximal Isometric Force (MIF) is the maximum force that can be exerted by a muscle or group of muscles in an isometric contraction. It is characterized by maintaining the highest possible tension without any joint movement, such as holding a heavy load in a static position, as in a maximal plank or wall sit.

Sub-maximal Isometric Force (sMIF) is a force exerted during an isometric contraction that is less than the muscle's maximum capacity. This is often used in endurance training or rehabilitation. Examples include maintaining a lighter load for an extended period or holding a partial squat position with moderate resistance.

Active Force Expressions

Active force expressions involve force production with movement, where muscles contract and cause joint motion. These are crucial for dynamic athletic activities where movement and power are key. Active Force Expressions are further divided into *Active and Reactive* categories.

Active Force Expressions

Active force expressions refer to the force generated through typical dynamic movements involving muscle contractions. This category includes both concentric (muscle shortening) and eccentric (muscle lengthening) contractions.

MDF is traditionally associated with the concept of one-repetition maximum (1RM), as mentioned in Chapter 1. This is the greatest amount of force generated during a dynamic muscle contraction, and it's typically seen in high-intensity movements, such as the maximum force exerted during a heavy lift, like a deadlift or a squat.

MEF is the highest force output generated in a very short period, and it is critical for movements requiring explosive power, like a sprinter pushing off the blocks, or a shot putter releasing the shot. It represents the optimal relationship between force and velocity across the entire load spectrum on the *force-velocity curve*, also known as *maximum power*.

Specific Task Force is the force applied in specific movements where efficiency, technique, and sustained effort are prioritized over sheer power, such as a marathon runner maintaining a consistent pace, or a tennis player executing a precise serve. It is crucial to understand the values of this expression, as it represents the goal that every trainer or coach aims to enhance.

Reactive Force Expressions

Reactive force expressions involve force generation in response to external stimuli, typically through quick, elastic responses, involving a rapid stretch-shortening cycle (SSC). This is crucial for activities requiring agility, reflexes, and explosive movements. It involves neuromuscular mechanisms that enable the production of the highest levels of force, as well as the ability to generate it rapidly.

Reactive Maximum Dynamic Force (rMDF) in the context of reactive expressions refers to the maximum force produced during quick, reactive movements, such as the force generated during the push-off phase of a rebound jump in basketball.

Reactive Maximum Explosive Force (rMEF) is the explosive force generated in response to external forces, often seen in plyometric exercises. An example of this is the force produced during the take-off in a depth jump.

Specific Task Force (Useful Force) is the force applied during specific reactive tasks where precision and timing are crucial, typically in sports requiring rapid direction changes or speed adjustments. For example, the force exerted by a soccer player when quickly changing direction in response to an opponent's movement is a specific task force.

ERF involves the generation of explosive force in response to a reactive stimulus, such as a quick stretch followed by an immediate contraction, The explosive force exerted during a plyometric box jump is an example of this, where the stretch-shortening cycle is rapidly engaged.

ERRF refers to the combination of explosive force and reflexive action, where the body reacts not only to a mechanical stimulus but also to a reflexive neural input. This is critical in situations requiring immediate, powerful responses to sudden changes, such as a volleyball player reacting to a quick spike and immediately jumping to block, combining reflex action with explosive force.

These classifications of force expressions provide a foundational framework for developing precise and effective training methods and programs tailored to specific needs, whether in strength and conditioning, physical therapy, or any other area within the field of sports science.

In strength and conditioning, programs can be meticulously tailored to enhance specific aspects of force production, such as boosting explosive power, dynamic strength, or reactive agility. For instance, an athlete looking to improve their sprinting power might focus on maximizing dynamic and explosive force expressions through a combination of targeted resistance training and plyometric exercises (González-Badillo et al., 2022). These methods are designed to increase the athlete's ability to generate force quickly, directly translating to improved sprint performance.

On the other hand, in physical therapy, rehabilitation programs can be precisely designed to restore and improve specific types of force expression, such as rebuilding isometric strength after an injury or enhancing reactive force for better functional movement. For example, a patient recovering from a knee injury might start with sub-maximal isometric exercises to safely rebuild stability and strength in the affected area. Once a solid foundation is established, the program could then progress to include reactive drills aimed at improving agility and restoring confidence in the patient's ability to move dynamically (Kraemer & Nitka, 2023).

These specific approaches in both strength and conditioning and physical therapy highlight the importance of understanding and applying the appropriate force expressions to meet the unique needs of everyone, whether the goal is peak athletic performance or effective rehabilitation. By focusing on the specific demands of each context, practitioners can create programs that not only address immediate needs but also contribute to long-term success and resilience.

Introducing the Concepts of Pushing and Holding

A novel and increasingly significant concept in both training and rehabilitation is the integration of traditional classifications of force expressions—such as dynamic, explosive, and reactive forces—with the fundamental actions of holding and pushing. These two basic muscle actions provide a deeper understanding of how force is applied and controlled in various movements. Holding and pushing are often seen as the foundation of all motor tasks, representing different forms of isometric contractions, each with unique characteristics and implications for training, rehabilitation, and performance (Schaefer & Bittmann, 2021).

Holding actions involve maintaining a static position against an external force, which is critical for building stability and postural control. For example, holding a plank position requires isometric contractions that engage the core and other stabilizing muscles, making it essential in both athletic training and rehabilitation settings. This type of force expression is crucial in sports that require prolonged stability under load, such as gymnastics or weightlifting, as well as in rehabilitation programs where restoring joint stability and muscular endurance is the primary goal.

Pushing actions, on the other hand, involve generating force to move or resist movement, often seen in dynamic efforts such as pushing a weight or accelerating the body during a sprint. Pushing represents a more active application of force, where the emphasis is on overcoming resistance and generating motion. This action is fundamental in sports where explosive power and quick force application are crucial, such as in football or basketball. In rehabilitation, pushing actions can be progressively introduced to restore functional strength and encourage muscle activation patterns that are critical for dynamic movement.

By integrating the concepts of holding and pushing into the traditional classification of force expressions, specialists can develop more nuanced and effective training and rehabilitation programs. This approach allows for a better understanding of how different types of force are applied in various contexts, leading to more targeted interventions that address specific needs, whether it's stabilizing a joint, improving explosive power, or restoring functional movement after an injury. This innovative perspective not only enriches the traditional methods but also provides a comprehensive framework that bridges the gap between static stability and dynamic power, ultimately enhancing performance and recovery across a wide range of activities.

Starting in the context of "isometric muscle actions," *holding* refers to the ability to resist an external force without changing the length of the muscle. This action is critical in scenarios where stability and endurance are required, such as maintaining a posture or position against a load. The Holding Isometric Muscle Action (HIMA) involves maintaining a static position by exerting just enough force to counterbalance an opposing force. This type of muscle action is akin to the concept of eccentric muscle contractions, where the muscle lengthens under tension, but in the case of HIMA, no actual lengthening occurs; instead, the muscle sustains the load without movement. This type of action is often associated with a faster onset of muscle fatigue due to the higher metabolic demands placed on the muscle to maintain the static position.

On the other hand, *pushing* in "isometric conditions," or pushing isometric muscle action (PIMA), involves exerting force against a stable resistance, where the muscle attempts to shorten but is prevented from doing so by an immovable object. PIMA is similar to concentric muscle contractions, where the muscle shortens under tension. In the context of PIMA, the muscle is engaged in a continuous effort to push or pull against resistance, which, while not resulting in visible movement, requires the muscle to generate and maintain force actively. This form of isometric action is typically associated with greater force endurance compared to HIMA, as the muscle is better supported by its own mechanical structure during the effort.

The distinction between these two forms of isometric muscle action is significant because it suggests different neuromuscular and physiological responses depending on whether the muscle is in a holding or pushing mode. Research, including the work of Schaefer and Bittmann (2017), has shown that muscles tend to fatigue more quickly during holding isometric actions compared to pushing ones. This is hypothesized to be due to the greater complexity of neural control strategies required during HIMA, as well as the potential for quicker metabolic fatigue in muscle fibers that are under continuous tension without the benefit of movement. For example, athletes who require prolonged static strength, such as gymnasts or wrestlers, might benefit from training that emphasizes holding isometric actions to improve their endurance and stability. Conversely, those engaged in activities that involve sustained pushing or pulling against resistance, such as weightlifting or rock climbing, might focus on pushing isometric actions to enhance their ability to generate and maintain force.

The differentiation between holding and pushing isometric muscle actions adds a layer of specificity to the understanding of muscle performance under static conditions. By recognizing the unique demands and benefits of each type of action, practitioners can better tailor their approaches to training and rehabilitation, ensuring that the exercises prescribed are optimally aligned with the desired outcomes.

In "dynamic actions," the concept of *holding* is often associated with the ability to stabilize certain parts of the body while other parts are in motion. This stabilization is crucial in maintaining balance, posture, and control during complex movements. For instance, when performing a squat, the muscles around the torso and core engage in a dynamic form of holding to stabilize the spine and pelvis, allowing the legs to perform the concentric (pushing) and eccentric (lowering) phases of the squat effectively. This dynamic holding, sometimes referred to as *dynamic stabilization*, ensures that the body's alignment and posture are maintained, thereby preventing injury and maximizing the efficiency of the movement.

Dynamic holding also plays a critical role in sports that require sudden changes of direction, such as basketball or soccer. Here, the ability to dynamically stabilize the body—essentially holding certain positions or joints steady while preparing for the next movement—can be the difference between a smooth transition and a loss of balance or control. For example, when a soccer player decelerates before a sharp turn, the muscles around the knees and hips must dynamically hold the joints in a stable position to prepare for the explosive push-off that follows.

Pushing in "dynamic actions" involves the active generation of force to move the body or an object. This force production is central to nearly all athletic movements, from sprinting and jumping to lifting and throwing. In dynamic contexts, pushing is typically associated with concentric muscle actions, where the muscle shortens as it generates force. However, in a dynamic environment, *pushing* also encompasses the transition from eccentric (lengthening) to concentric actions, particularly in activities that require rapid or explosive movements.

For instance, in a sprint, the *pushing action* occurs during the drive phase where the athlete propels themselves forward by pushing off the ground with each step. This *pushing action* is not only about generating force but also about doing so with the correct timing and coordination to maximize speed and efficiency. The ability to push dynamically is also crucial in powerlifting, where the athlete must push the barbell away from their body during the bench press or clean and jerk, integrating both strength and speed to achieve the lift.

Figure 2.1 provides a concise summary of the relationship between load percentages and movement velocity, illustrating how different types of force expressions—specifically Holding (H) and Pushing (P)—correlate with various training intensities. The graph is divided into categories representing specific muscle actions and force production methods, with particular emphasis on explosive maximum force (EMF), MDF, and other key concepts in strength training. This visualization helps to clearly differentiate how holding and pushing actions interact with load and velocity to optimize training outcomes.

The classification of force expressions considering this new concept is outlined next. This approach aims to integrate the traditional categories with the new understanding, offering a more comprehensive frame for analyzing and applying different types of force, or expressions, in various training and performance contexts.

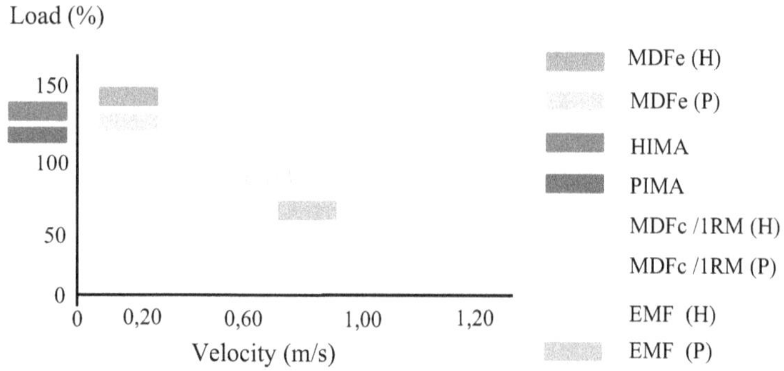

Figure 2.1 Key variables in strength training and their applications.

1. **Passive Force Expressions** involve force production without movement, where muscles generate tension but do not change length. These expressions are crucial for stability, posture, and maintaining positions against resistance.

    - **Maximal Isometric Force (MIF)**:
    - **Holding Action (HIMA)** is primarily holding, where the muscle maintains tension without any external movement, for example, holding a heavy weight in a static position, such as in a maximal plank or wall sit.
    - **Pushing Action (PIMA)** is typically associated with dynamic movements, but pushing can also occur isometrically when exerting force against an immovable object. Pushing against a wall or an immovable bar in an isometric squat are such examples.

- **Sub-maximal Isometric Force**:

    - **Holding Action** is sustaining a sub-maximal level of tension over time, often seen in postural or stabilizing activities. Examples include holding a lighter load for an extended period or maintaining a partial squat position with moderate resistance.
    - **Pushing Actions**, similar to maximal isometric pushing, but with less intensity, are used to build endurance and stability, in exercises like lightly pushing against a resistance band or a stable surface over an extended time.

Active Force Expressions

Active force expressions involve force production with movement, where muscles contract and cause joint motion. These are essential for dynamic athletic activities and are further divided into active and reactive force expressions.

Active Force

Active Force refers to the force generated through typical dynamic movements involving muscle contractions, including both concentric (muscle shortening) and eccentric (muscle lengthening).

MDF:

- **Pushing Actions** focus on pushing against resistance during movement, such as during a heavy lift, like the maximum force exerted during a deadlift or squat.
- **Holding Actions**, while less common in dynamic actions, are brief moments where holding force is required, such as at the peak of a lift before lowering, when a lifter briefly holds the barbell at the top of a deadlift.

MEF:

- **Pushing Action**: Pushing force is rapidly applied to generate movement, which is critical in explosive tasks, like when a sprinter pushes off the blocks or a shot putter releases the shot.
- **Holding Action**: Holding is often minimized in explosive movements, but it can occur in preparation for the explosive action when athletes hold the starting position before an explosive sprint.

Specific Task Force (Useful Force):

- **Pushing Action**: Pushing is controlled and often sustained over the duration of the task. A marathon runner maintaining a consistent pace is a good example of this.
- **Holding Action**: Holding plays a role in stabilizing or preparing for more precise, controlled movements; for example, a tennis player holding a ready stance before executing a precise serve.

Reactive Force

Reactive force involves force generation in response to external stimuli, typically through quick, elastic responses involving a rapid stretch-shortening cycle (SSC). This is crucial for activities requiring agility, reflexes, and explosive movements.

rMDF:

- **Pushing Action**: Pushing force is applied rapidly in response to an external force, such as the force generated during the push-off phase of a rebound jump in basketball.
- **Holding Action**: Brief holding phases may occur in reactive scenarios, such as stabilizing before or after a reactive movement, for example briefly holding a defensive stance before reacting in a basketball game.

rMDF:

- **Pushing Action**: The focus is on explosive pushing off a surface or against resistance, such as the force produced during a depth jump take-off.
- **Holding Action**: Holding is usually minimized in explosive movements, but may occur briefly before the explosive phase, for example, holding a crouch position before exploding upward in a jump.

Specific Task Force (Useful Force):

- **Pushing Action**: Pushing is applied dynamically in response to external stimuli, focusing on specific task efficiency, such as the force exerted by a soccer player when quickly changing direction.
- **Holding Action**: Holding is used to stabilize or prepare for a quick directional change, for example, holding a balanced position before executing a rapid pivot.

ERF:

- **Pushing Action**: The primary action is pushing off from the ground or an object explosively, like the explosive force exerted during a plyometric box jump.
- **Holding Action**: Brief holding phases may be used to stabilize before or after the explosive action, such as holding balance on landing after a box jump.

ERRF:

- **Pushing Action**: Rapid and powerful pushing movements in response to a reflexive stimulus. An example is a volleyball player reacting to a quick spike and immediately jumping to block.
- **Holding Action**: Holding occurs as a stabilizing action, often after the reflexive movement, to prepare for the next action, for example stabilizing the body immediately after landing from a reactive jump.

Integration and Interplay of Force Expressions in Real-World Movements

Pure movements that involve only one type of force expression are exceedingly rare. Most movements, especially those involved in sports, physical activities, and daily tasks, are complex and involve a combination of different force expressions. This complexity arises because real-world actions typically require the body to adapt and respond to varying demands, combining different types of force to achieve a specific goal.

For example, a single athletic movement like a jump shot in basketball involves a mixture of force expressions:

1. Passive Force Expression: Holding force may be used to stabilize the body before the jump, as the athlete gathers power and prepares for the movement.
2. Active Force Expression: As the athlete begins to jump, there is a dynamic push-off that involves maximum dynamic force to propel the body upward.
3. Reactive Force Expression: Upon landing, the body must quickly react to absorb the impact and stabilize, potentially involving reactive and reflexive force expressions.

Similarly, during a simple daily task like lifting a box:

1. Passive force may be engaged as the individual holds the box in a stationary position.
2. Active force is utilized to lift the box dynamically from the ground.
3. Reactive force may come into play if the person needs to adjust their grip or stance suddenly to maintain balance.

The Importance of Recognizing Mixed Expressions in Training and Therapy

Understanding that most movements involve a mix of force expressions is vital for developing effective training programs and rehabilitation protocols (McGill, 2015). By acknowledging the interplay of different force expressions, trainers can design more comprehensive and realistic training programs. These programs should not only target isolated muscle actions but also consider how these actions integrate into more complex, functional movements. This approach ensures that athletes develop the strength, power, and coordination needed for real-world performance (Siff & Verkhoshansky, 1999).

In rehabilitation, recognizing mixed-force expressions allows physical therapists to create more effective recovery plans. For instance, after an injury, a patient might first need to focus on regaining isometric holding strength before gradually reintroducing dynamic and reactive movements (Kibler & Livingston, 2001). This progression mirrors the natural complexity of human movement, helping the patient return to full functionality more efficiently.

Depending on the task, exercise, or gesture being performed, the emphasis on different force expressions can be adjusted. For example, in sports where quick change of direction (COD) are frequent, more focus might be placed on developing reactive and reflexive forces. In contrast, in activities requiring sustained power output, such as rowing or cycling, training might focus more on dynamic and specific task forces.

Key Variables in Strength Training: Measurement and Manipulation

The understanding and manipulation of basic physical variables are fundamental to designing precise and effective training programs. These variables, such as force, velocity, acceleration, and work, are intrinsic to every movement or position, collectively determining the forces and outcomes involved in any exercise or physical activity. By accurately measuring and adjusting these variables, trainers, coaches, and physical therapists can create targeted stimuli to achieve specific training goals, whether they relate to strength, power, endurance, or rehabilitation (Newton & Kraemer, 1994).

These basic variables serve as independent variables in the context of training interventions. For instance, force (measured as load) and velocity (the speed of movement) can be manipulated to create specific training effects, such as increasing muscle mass or improving explosive power. However, these variables can also function as dependent variables, as they respond to the adjustments made during training. For example, increasing the load in a squat not only requires more force but also influences the speed at which the movement can be performed, thus impacting power output and overall training efficacy (Cormie et al., 2011).

Understanding how these variables interact and how to measure or manipulate them is crucial for designing effective training programs and analyzing performance. Mastery of these variables allows coaches, trainers, and therapists to create precise stimuli tailored to specific goals, such as enhancing strength, increasing power, improving endurance, or facilitating recovery. This detailed approach ensures that each aspect of training is grounded in a solid understanding of the underlying physics, leading to more effective and efficient outcomes (Siff & Verkhoshansky, 1999).

Moreover, viewing these variables as both independent and dependent enables professionals to better control and measure the effects of their interventions, facilitating a more scientific and individualized approach to training. This dual perspective provides deeper insight into how different training methods impact the body, optimizing training regimens for a variety of populations and objectives.

Table 2.1 provides a comprehensive overview of the essential physical variables involved in strength training. It outlines their definitions, units of measurement, formulas, and practical applications in designing and refining training programs. This table serves as a useful reference for understanding how these variables can be manipulated to achieve specific training outcomes, such as increasing muscle mass, enhancing power, or improving functional performance.

In summary, this chapter provides a thorough exploration of the various expressions of force, integrating traditional concepts with contemporary approaches. The chapter also explains the complex interplay between different types of force expressions, emphasizing that real-world movements often involve a combination of these expressions, a crucial factor in the design of training programs needed for enhanced performance. Finally, an overview of key variables, outlining their definitions, units of measurement, formulas, and practical applications provides a quick reference.

Table 2.1 Key variables in strength training and their applications

Variable	*Definition*	*Units*	*Formula*	*Application*
Force (F)	A push or pull exerted on an object	Newton (N)	$F = m \times a$	Manipulating force alters the intensity of exercises and the resistance the muscles work against.
Mass (m)	The amount of matter in an object	Kilograms (kg)	N/A	Adjusting mass directly affects the resistance in strength training exercises.
Acceleration (a)	The rate of change of velocity of an object	m/s^2	$a = \Delta v/\Delta t$	A crucial application in explosive movements as increasing acceleration requires greater force.
Velocity (v)	The speed of something in a given direction	m/s	$v = \Delta x/\Delta t$	This is a key factor in power development; higher-velocity movements enhance performance.
Displacement (x)	The change in position of an object	Meters (m)	N/A	Modifying displacement changes the range of motion, affecting mechanical demand.
Work (W)	The amount of energy transferred by a force over a distance	Joules (J)	$W = F \times d \times \cos(\theta)$	Increasing work by increasing force or distance can lead to greater strength gains.
Energy (E)	The capacity to do work	Joules (J)	KE: $1/2\ mv^2$, PE: $m \times g \times h$	Understanding energy dynamics aids in designing programs that balance kinetic and potential energy.
Power (P)	The rate at which work is done or energy is transferred	Watts (W)	$P = W/t$ or $P = F \times v$	Power is crucial in explosive movements; manipulating it can optimize strength and speed.
Momentum (p)	The quantity of motion an object has	kg·m/s	$p = m \times v$	This is vital for maximizing efficiency in movements requiring quick direction changes or impacts.
Impulse (J)	Change in momentum resulting from a force applied over time	N·s	$J = F \times \Delta t$	The key for altering motion quickly, impulse is essential in sports requiring rapid starts and stops.
Torque (τ)	A measure of the force that can cause an object to rotate	N·m	$\tau = F \times r \times \sin(\theta)$	Adjusting torque changes the focus of exercises and is essential for rotational movements.

References

Cormie, P., McGuigan, M. R., & Newton, R. U. (2011). Developing maximal neuromuscular power: Part 1—biological basis of maximal power production. *Sports Medicine*, *41*(1), 17–38.

Enoka, R. M. (2008). *Neuromechanics of human movement* (4th ed.). Human Kinetics.

González-Badillo, J. J., Sánchez-Medina, L., Ribas-Serna, J., & Rodríguez-Rosell, D. (2022). Toward a new paradigm in resistance training by means of velocity monitoring: A critical and challenging narrative. *Sports Medicine—Open*, *8*(118). https://doi.org/10.1186/s40798-022-00513-z

Kibler, W. B., & Livingston, B. (2001). Closed-chain rehabilitation for upper and lower extremities. *JAAOS-Journal of the American Academy of Orthopaedic Surgeons*, *9*(6), 412–421.

Kraemer, W. J., & Nitka, M. (2023). Choice of resistance used in an exercise: Simple to complex interactions. *Strength and Conditioning Journal*, *44*(4), 123–126.

Lieber, R. L. (2010). *Skeletal muscle structure, function, and plasticity* (3rd ed.). Lippincott Williams & Wilkins.

McGill, S. (2015). *Low back disorders: Evidence-based prevention and rehabilitation*. Human Kinetics.

Newton, R. U., & Kraemer, W. J. (1994). Developing explosive muscular power: Implications for a mixed methods training strategy. *Strength & Conditioning Journal*, *16*(5), 20–31.

Schaefer, L. V., & Bittmann, F. N. (2017). Are there two forms of isometric muscle action? Results of the experimental study support a distinction between a holding and a pushing isometric muscle function. *BMC Sports Science, Medicine and Rehabilitation*, *9*, 1–13.

Schaefer, L. V., & Bittmann, F. N. (2021). Paired personal interaction reveals objective differences between pushing and holding isometric muscle action. *PLoS One*, *16*(5), e0238331.

Siff, M. C., & Verkhoshansky, Y. V. (1999). *Supertraining* (5th ed.). Denver: Supertraining Institute.

Tous-Fajardo, J. (1999). *Nuevas tendencias en fuerza y musculación*. Editorial Hispano Europea.

Vittori, C. (1990). El entrenamiento de la fuerza para el sprint. *Red: Revista de Entrenamiento Deportivo*, *4*(3), 2–8.

Zatsiorsky, V. M., & Prilutsky, B. I. (2012). *Biomechanics of skeletal muscles*. Human Kinetics.

3 Validity and Reliability of Evaluation with Functional Electromechanical Devices

Ángela Rodríguez-Perea and Ignacio J. Chirosa Rios

Introduction to Evaluation with FEMD

Functional electromechanical devices (FEMD) have emerged as a pivotal tool in the assessment of physical performance. These devices represent the convergence of mechanical engineering, computer science, and human physiology, offering unprecedented precision in evaluating various aspects of physical fitness. The evolution of FEMD from basic mechanical testing tools to sophisticated systems capable of real-time data processing reflects broader trends in technology and sports science.

The integration of FEMD into modern training and rehabilitation programs has brought about a paradigm shift in how evaluations are conducted. No longer reliant solely on subjective assessments or less precise methods, trainers and clinicians can now obtain objective data that can be used to tailor programs with remarkable specificity. This shift has made it possible to monitor progress with greater accuracy and to identify potential issues before they become serious problems.

The Importance of Evaluation in Physical Training and Rehabilitation

Historically, physical evaluation has played a crucial role in both athletic training and rehabilitation. Traditional methods often relied on manual measurements, basic tools like goniometers, and subjective observation, which, while useful, had significant limitations. The advent of FEMD technology has addressed many of these limitations by providing reliable, repeatable, and highly accurate data that can be used to make informed decisions.

In the realm of rehabilitation, accurate evaluation is especially critical. For patients recovering from injury, the ability to measure progress in terms of strength, range of motion, and endurance can significantly impact recovery outcomes. FEMD allows for the tracking of these metrics in real time, enabling therapists to adjust treatment protocols as needed.

DOI: 10.4324/9781003425182-4

The importance of evaluation extends beyond professional athletes and patients in rehabilitation. Individuals at all levels of fitness can benefit from understanding their physical capabilities, whether their goal is to improve overall health, increase athletic performance, or simply maintain functional mobility as they age. FEMD provides a comprehensive toolset for this purpose, making high-quality evaluation accessible to a broader population.

Before relying on any new technology, it is necessary to prove its validity and reliability to measure key metrics. To trust the outcomes, it is necessary to understand exactly what validity and reliability are, and how these metrics are tested.

Validity

The validation of a test/instrument can be classified into three categories: content validity, criterion validity, and construct validity. Content validity refers to how well the test/instrument contains the correct number of items, according to its intended purpose. For example, if the questionnaire used to measure anxiety truly assesses anxiety with each of its constituent items. To assess whether an item is correct, it is evaluated by experts in the field and is assessed using the content validity ratio (CVR) (Lawshe 1975). This index is calculated using the following formula, where *ne* is the number of experts who rate the item as essential, and *N* is the total number of experts evaluating it. The range of the CVR varies from −1 to 1.

$$CVR = \frac{n_e - N/2}{N/2}$$

Another type of coefficient used to measure content validity is the Kappa coefficient, which indicates the degree of agreement among raters and is employed to classify nominal variables. Additionally, Kendall's W concordance coefficient is used to assess the degree of agreement among experts and provides an overall evaluation of the test. Both coefficients range from 0 to 1. The intraclass correlation coefficient (ICC), which is a measure that evaluates the agreement among judges or experts in their item ratings or the relationship between the test/instrument to be validated, considered the gold standard and ranges from 0 to 1, can also be found. In the object of study of this book, the FEMD was validated with a linear encoder, considered the gold standard for measuring the velocity of displacement in the assessment of force, before being used to know the validity of its measurements in isokinetic mode (Rodriguez-Perea et al. 2021) (Figure 3.1). Another coefficient that can be used to study the relationship between two tests/instruments is the Pearson correlation coefficient. The closer this coefficient is to 1, the better the validity (W. G. Hopkins et al. 2009). If a more visual method of identifying the validity of the test/instrument is desired, Bland-Altman plots can be used, which indicate the

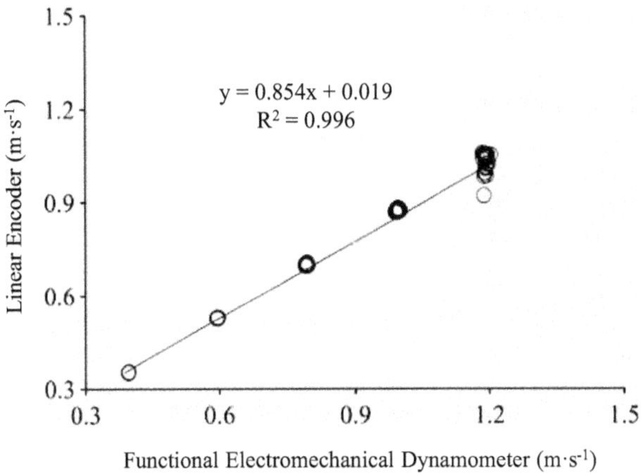

Figure 3.1 Validity of FEMD compared with linear encoder.

degree of difference between the two tests/instruments and the limits of agreement (Martin Bland and Altman 1986, 1995).

The criterion validity of a research test/instrument is established by correlating the scores obtained from applying the test/instrument with the scores obtained from another external criterion that is intended to be measured (Hernández Sampieri et al. 2014). An instrument is compared with another external instrument that has good validity. Within criterion validity, depending on the timing of the assessment, there is concurrent validity when the results are compared at the same moment or point in time, and predictive validity, which pertains to how accurately a test measures the criterion being evaluated and predicts it over time. Additionally, there is internal validity, used when evaluating a test to be used, and it is validated against a test that measures the same thing to determine how the test excludes alternative explanations for the measurements. External validity is used to validate a test against an external criterion.

In criterion validity, different coefficients are used, such as the Pearson correlation coefficient (for normally distributed variables, with values ranging from 1 to –1), Spearman correlation coefficient (for non-normally distributed variables, with values ranging from 1 to –1), simple linear regression (to predict criterion values from test scores), or the Kappa concordance coefficient. The choice of a particular coefficient depends on the nature of the data and the relationship between the test/instrument and the criterion.

In summary, when evaluating the criterion validity of a questionnaire created to assess anxiety with another previously validated anxiety questionnaire, the results from both tests should be similar to assert that the new questionnaire is valid. To provide a more relatable example in this context, if the speed at which a load moves using a new device is being assessed, it is necessary to have a previously validated device to determine the validity of the new one.

Construct validity is used to verify that a test or instrument truly measures the construct or trait it intends to measure. The construct is a measured variable that fits within a hypothesis, theory, or theoretical framework (Hernández Sampieri et al. 2014). It is assessed using the Kappa coefficient.

Therefore, for a test/instrument to be valid, it needs to possess the highest content, criterion, and construct validity to accurately evaluate the variable it aims to measure.

Reliability

Reliability is the consistency or stability of a measurement obtained in a test evaluated at different points in time. There are different methods to assess reliability, with the test-retest being the most widely used among researchers and trainers in this field. The recommended time interval between the two measurements varies from 2 to 14 days.

There are two types of reliability, relative reliability and absolute reliability. Relative reliability indicates how similar a participant's order is between test and retest for the group (Weir 2005), and absolute reliability refers to how an individual repeats the values obtained in a test at different times of assessment. The main problem with relative reliability is that it depends on the variability of the sample, whereas absolute reliability is related to the consistency of the score obtained individually (W. Hopkins 2000; W. G. Hopkins et al. 2009).

Relative Reliability

For the assessment of relative reliability, the ICC is used, which compares the variance between subjects with the total variance of the sample. Hopkins et al. (2009), classified the magnitude of the values of the ICC through a qualitative scale: values close to 0.1 are considered low reliability; 0.3, moderate; 0.5, high; 0.7, very high; and those close to 0.9, extremely high (W. G. Hopkins et al. 2009).

Absolute Reliability

Absolute reliability is measured with different errors or coefficients such as the standard error of measurement (SEM), the minimum detectable change (MDC), or the coefficient of variation (CV).

The SEM is an indicator of the lack of consistency between the values obtained in the test, with a high SEM value indicating low test reliability.

These measures were calculated as follows with a value of SEM $\leq$ 15% considered acceptable (Weir 2005):

$$\%SEM = \text{mean of the difference scores between 2 trials} \times 100/\text{mean of the first trial}$$

MDC refers to the smallest change in a variable that is statistically significant or surpasses the level of variability in the measurement. To estimate the MDC in a score that indicates a "real change" in 90% of participants, the MDC_{90} (del Corral et al. 2020) was calculated:

$$MDC_{90} = SEM \times \sqrt{2x1.65}.$$

CV is used to express the relative variability of a sample concerning the standard deviation and mean and to calculate:

$$CV = (sd/mean) \times 100.$$

The result is expressed as a percentage, and the absolute value can be calculated from the mean. A smaller CV indicates a more reliable measurement.

Factors Affecting Validity and Reliability

Several factors can affect the validity of a test/instrument. First of these is the response bias, which refers to a participant's tendency not to accurately reflect their real thoughts or capabilities. Another factor is sample bias, where the sample evaluated does not represent the population of interest. Additionally, changes in the construct over time, referring to changes in the construct being measured, can affect validity.

Factors that can affect reliability are dependent on test development. It's important to consider all conditions when conducting a test to replicate them accurately. Therefore, one factor is variability in measurement conditions, including environmental factors like temperature, noise, or other environmental factors. It's also crucial to control who administers the test, ensuring it's the same person to maintain reliability. Another aspect to control is the instructions given for the test. In this field of study, it's essential to keep all these factors stable and standardize protocols as much as possible to prevent errors that might reduce test reliability.

Strategies to Improve Validity and Reliability

To enhance the validity of tests, various strategies can be implemented. For content validity, content experts can contribute, pilot tests can be conducted to gather information, correction of confusing items, finally the items to be evaluated must be defined and reviewed to ensure they evaluate the intended metrics. In the case of criterion validity, it's essential to establish strong, previously validated external criteria to evaluate test validity and assess the relationship between test measures and external measures to determine concurrent or predictive validity. For construct validity, consider the construct used to accurately reflect the variable being evaluated and ensure that both measurement objectives and goals are related to the construct definition.

Regarding reliability, as mentioned earlier, standardizing the evaluation process and, if necessary, creating a step-by-step manual for the procedures are crucial. Additionally, evaluators should be trained to perform evaluations in a standardized manner, and all environmental conditions should be controlled. The more the variables that can affect the assessments are controlled, the better the validity and reliability will be. Among the variables that can affect the test are the time of day when the test is performed, the instructions given to the participants, the fatigue produced by the test, where the participant is asked to focus their attention, the order of the tests, the fatigue of the subject, the nutritional status, and the warm-up (McGuigan 2020).

Practical Application of Validity and Reliability

The practical application of validity and reliability in this field of study is essential to identify which test to use when measuring a variable or when creating new valid and reliable tests/instruments. These concepts are relevant both when evaluating an athlete or a patient and when making clinical decisions, such as return-to-play after an injury.

Reliability of Functional Electromechanical Dynamometer Test

The FEMD is a novel device and therefore it has been necessary to create assessment protocols and study its reliability. Numerous studies have evaluated the reliability of different tests and compared different assessment conditions to find out which is the most reliable (Table 3.1).

To enhance the reliability of a test or assessment conducted with FEMD, it is essential to establish a standardized protocol. The following considerations should be considered:

1. Conduct a pilot test of all processes involved in the evaluation beforehand.
2. Ensure that participants in the study are familiar with the specific requirements of the test, providing explanations tailored to their level of understanding.
3. For individuals with injuries or age-related physical deterioration, implement a preliminary adaptation process. For instance, in cases of limb injury,

Table 3.1 Reliability of functional electromechanical dynamometer test

	Exercise/movement	*Device*	*Condition assessment*	*ICC*	*CV (%)*
Lower Body	Hip abduction	Haefni Health v.1.0	Isometric	0.94	5.64
	Squat	FEMD (Dynasystem, Model Research, Granada, Spain)	Tonic: incremental test	>0.95	<8.48
	Mid-thigh pull	FEMD (Dynasystem, Model Research, Granada, Spain)	Isometric	0.94	2.51
	Knee Extension	FEMD (Dynasystem, Model Research, Granada, Spain)	Isometric	>0.95	<8.63
			Vibratory Isometric	>0.97	<8.23
Upper Body	Shoulder External/ internal rotation	FEMD (Dynasystem, Model Research, Granada, Spain)	Isokinetic (0.6 ms)	>0.87	<6.87
	Shoulder Flexion	Myoquality M1 (Myoquality Solutions, Granada, Spain)	Isokinetic (0.8 ms)	>0.80	<15.88
	Shoulder Extension			>0.76	<19.63
	Shoulder Abduction			>0.81	<15.91
	Shoulder Adduction			>0.85	<18.76
	Bench Press		Isometric	0.99	4.65
		FEMD (Dynasystem, Model Research, Granada, Spain)	Vibratory Isometric	0.98	<5.02
	Row		Isometric	0.92	9.61
			Vibratory Isometric	>0.95	<7.17
Trunk	Flexors	FEMD (Dynasystem, Model Research, Granada, Spain)	Isokinetic 0.15 ms	0.82–0.85	<7.67
	Extensors			0.81–0.85	<11.33
	Rotators		Isokinetic 0.40 ms	0.85–0.89	<10.21
Functional Test	Sit to stand	FEMD (Dynasystem, Model Research, Granada, Spain)	Tonic: 3 loads	>0.98	<6.04
Sports Specific Test	Swing Eccentric Hamstring Exercise	FEMD (Dynasystem, Model Research, Granada, Spain)	Isokinetic (0.20;0.40; 0.60 ms)	0.87–0.91	<5.85
	Unilateral pullover	FEMD (Dynasystem, Model Research, Granada, Spain)	Tonic: incremental test	0.83–0.96	<8.99
	Standing lift			0.85–0.97	<10.93
	Step forward			0.87–0.93	<11.57
	Defensive two-step test	FEMD (Dynasystem, Model Research, Granada, Spain)	Tonic: 15% BW	0.79	1.34

test the unaffected side first to establish a baseline and reduce apprehension or reluctance to perform the test with the injured side.

4. Clearly define and adhere to a specific warm-up procedure appropriate for the mode of use being employed.
5. Provide precise instructions to the participant, using consistent language that clearly communicates the required actions during the test.
6. Have well-rehearsed protocols in place to anticipate and manage potential challenges, such as where and how to secure equipment.
7. Manage all potential mechanical risks to avoid contingencies, including securing equipment to the wall, understanding the capacities of external materials used, and assessing their wear and tear (e.g., ropes, pulleys).
8. Ensure that all equipment is prepared, with all accessories checked and ready for use.
9. Consider the entire evaluation protocol, including how and where to position oneself, the initial and final positions, etc.

The reliability of different tests for the assessment of the lower body has been extensively studied. Cerda Vega et al. (2018) assessed hip abduction strength in three positions (side lying, standing and supine) and concluded that the supine position was the most reliable with an ICC of 0.94 and a CV of 5.64% (Vega et al. 2018). Del-Cuerpo et al. (2023) assessed the reliability of squat exercise with different outcome variables such as range of motion, mean and peak dynamic strength, mean and peak velocity, mean and peak power, work, and momentum, and obtained high reliability for all measured variables (ICC > 0.95; CV < 8.48%) (del-Cuerpo et al. 2023). Furthermore, reliability was assessed for the mid-thigh pull in the isometric mode for 10 seconds, with very high reliability for peak force (ICC = 0.94; CV = 2.51%) (Baena-Raya et al. 2021). Another study demonstrated high reliability for unilateral knee extension in the isometric mode (ICC > 0.95; CV < 8.63) and in isometric mode with vibration at two different intensities: 20 Hz (ICC > 0.97; CV < 8.23) and 40 Hz (ICC = 0.98; CV < 4.93) (Andrades-Ramírez et al. 2024).

In the upper body, reliability has been determined for all shoulder movements. The external and internal rotator strength of the shoulder was assessed, and different velocities (0.3 and 0.6 ms^{-1}) were compared, and high reliability was obtained for both velocities (ICC > 0.81; CV < 8.27%), with the 0.6 ms^{-1} velocity being the most reliable (ICC > 0.87; CV < 6.87%) (Martinez-Garcia et al. 2020). Additionally, reliability was assessed for flexion, extension, abduction, and adduction at a speed of 0.80 ms^{-1}, both for peak force and for average force, and the reliability was very high to extremely high for all movements on concentric and eccentric strength measurements (ICC > 0.76; CV < 19.63%) (García-Buendía et al. 2024). Moreover, a study analyzed the seated bench press, demonstrating high reliability in the isometric mode (ICC = 0.99; CV = 4.65%) and in isometric mode with vibration at two different intensities: 20 Hz (ICC = 0.98; CV = 4.95) and 40 Hz (ICC = 0.98; CV = 5.02%) and bilateral seated row with high reliability in the isometric mode (ICC = 0.92; CV = 9.61) and isometric mode with vibration at two different intensities: 20 Hz (ICC = 0.95; CV = 8.38) and 40 Hz (ICC = 0.96; CV = 7.17) (Andrades-Ramírez et al. 2024).

In the trunk, reliability studies have been conducted for trunk flexors, extensors, and rotators. Different velocities and ranges of movement were compared. In trunk flexors, the most reliable condition was the low velocity (0.15 ms^{-1}) and in short ranges of movement, obtaining high reliability (ICC = 0.82–0.85; CV = 6.82%–7.67%), as in extensors (ICC = 0.81–0.85; CV = 9.52%–11.33%) (Rodriguez-Perea et al. 2019; Reyes-Ferrada et al. 2022). For the assessment of the rotators, two exercises were compared (Horizontal and Low Cable Woodchop) at two velocities and it was found that the horizontal exercise at the low velocity provided more reliable data (ICC = 0.85–0.89; CV = 9.52%–11.33%) (Rodríguez-Perea et al. 2023).

The reliability of functional tests such as sit-to-stand with different loads (5, 10, and 15 kg) have also been studied, and they obtained high reliability for all peak strength conditions (ICC > 0.98; CV < 6.04%) (Jerez-Mayorga et al. 2021).

Also, reliability has been studied in specific gestures of different sports. In the case of football players, the reliability of an eccentric swing exercise for hamstrings at three velocities (0.20, 0.40, and 0.60 ms^{-1}) was assessed and the slowest velocity (0.20 ms^{-1}) was found to be the most reliable (ICC = 0.91; CV = 4.66%) (Sánchez-Sánchez et al. 2021). In professional handball players, the reliability of three unilateral exercises pullover, standing lift, and step forward was studied and obtained a high reliability (ICC= 0.83–0.97; CV = 3.90%–11.57%) (Morenas-Aguilar et al. 2023). Another study determined the reliability of a two-step defensive test in professional handball players in tonic mode with two loads relative to each player's body weight (15% and 30%). It was found that the 15% body weight load was more reliable (ICC = 0.79; CV = 1.34%) (Chirosa-Ríos et al. 2022).

In summary, the reliability and validity of FEMDs have been verified in many different studies, for many muscle groups in many different sports. It is time to highlight the advantages and key metrics that this type of evaluation provides and discuss how it can inform training and rehabilitation decisions.

Key Metrics in FEMD Evaluation

Maximum Strength

Maximum strength is a fundamental aspect of physical fitness, influencing everything from basic daily activities to elite athletic performance. FEMD provides several methods for assessing maximum strength, each with its own advantages. These include:

- One-Repetition Maximum (1RM)
- Dynamic Maximum Strength

- Isometric Maximum Strength
- Explosive Strength
- Rate of Force Development (RFD)
- Peak Power

Velocity and Speed

Velocity is another critical factor in physical performance, particularly in sports that require fast, dynamic movements. FEMD allows for precise measurement of velocity, providing insights into both performance and fatigue, including:

- Peak Velocity
- Velocity Loss

Endurance and Fatigue Resistance

Muscular endurance and fatigue resistance are crucial for sustained physical activity, whether in sports, work, or daily life. FEMD provides tools for measuring these attributes, offering insights into how muscles perform over time, including:

- Force Decay
- Repetitions Until Fatigue

Balance and Symmetry

Balance and symmetry in muscle strength are important for both performance and injury prevention. FEMD allows for the precise measurement of these attributes, helping to identify and correct imbalances.

- Bilateral Balance
- Agonist/Antagonist Ratios

Range of motion (ROM) is a key component of flexibility and mobility, affecting everything from basic movements to complex athletic maneuvers. FEMD provides tools for measuring ROM with high accuracy.

- Total ROM
- Consistency in ROM

Specific Performance Metrics

In addition to the general metrics discussed earlier, FEMD can measure specific performance metrics that provide deeper insights into an individual's capabilities.

- Kinetic Patterns
- Force-Velocity Profiles

Advanced Evaluation Protocols with FEMD

Designing an Effective Evaluation Protocol

Designing an effective evaluation protocol with FEMD involves several steps, each aimed at ensuring that the data collected is accurate, reliable, and relevant to the individual's goals.

- **Step-by-Step Guide to Designing Custom Evaluation Protocols**: The first step in designing an evaluation protocol is to define the specific goals of the evaluation. This might include assessing maximum strength, explosive power, endurance, or other attributes. Once the goals are defined, the appropriate metrics and exercises can be selected. The protocol should be tailored to the individual's needs and capabilities, considering factors such as their fitness level, experience, and any existing injuries.
- **Considerations for Different Populations (Athletes, Elderly, Rehabilitation)**: Different populations have different needs and considerations when it comes to evaluation. For athletes, the focus might be on optimizing performance and identifying areas for improvement. For the elderly, the focus might be on maintaining mobility and preventing falls. In rehabilitation settings, the goal might be to assess recovery progress and adjust treatment plans accordingly. FEMD can be used to design protocols that meet the specific needs of each population.

Familiarization and Warm-Up Procedures

Familiarization and warm-up are critical components of the evaluation process, helping to ensure accurate measurements and reduce the risk of injury.

- **Best Practices for Ensuring Accurate Measurements**: Familiarization involves introducing the individual to the FEMD equipment and exercises to reduce variability in performance due to unfamiliarity. A proper warm-up is also essential, as it prepares the muscles and joints for maximum effort tests. The warm-up should be specific to the exercises being performed and should include both general and specific movements.
- **Case Studies on the Impact of Warm-Up on Evaluation Outcomes**: Research has shown that a proper warm-up can significantly impact the outcomes of an evaluation. For example, a study on athletes found that those who performed a specific warm-up protocol before a 1RM test were able to lift significantly more weight than those who did not.

Conducting Evaluations

The actual process of conducting evaluations with FEMD involves several important steps, each aimed at ensuring that the data collected is accurate and reliable.

- **Advanced Techniques for Data Collection and Analysis**: FEMD allows for the collection of a wide range of data during an evaluation, including force, velocity, power, and more. Advanced techniques for data collection might include the use of high-speed cameras, motion capture systems, and specialized software for analyzing complex data sets. The goal is to obtain the most accurate and detailed data possible, which can then be used to inform training decisions.

Post-evaluation Analysis

After the evaluation, the data collected must be carefully analyzed to extract meaningful insights.

- **Using Software Tools for Data Analysis**: There are a variety of software tools available for analyzing FEMD data, ranging from basic spreadsheet programs to specialized software for biomechanical analysis. These tools can be used to process large data sets, identify trends, and generate reports that summarize the key findings of the evaluation.
- **Interpretation of Complex Data Sets: A Guide for Practitioners**: Interpreting the data collected during an FEMD evaluation can be challenging, particularly when dealing with complex data sets that include multiple variables. Practitioners should have a solid understanding of the underlying principles of biomechanics and statistics, as well as experience in using the relevant software tools.

Re-evaluation and Longitudinal Tracking

Periodic re-evaluations are an important part of any training or rehabilitation program, allowing for the monitoring of progress and the adjustment of protocols as needed.

- **Designing Long-Term Evaluation Programs**: Long-term evaluation programs involve regular re-evaluations at set intervals, such as every few weeks or months. These programs can be used to track progress over time, identify trends, and adjust training or rehabilitation protocols. FEMD allows for the precise tracking of multiple metrics, making it an ideal tool for long-term evaluation.

- **Integrating Continuous Monitoring with Periodic Re-evaluations**: In addition to periodic re-evaluations, continuous monitoring can provide valuable insights into an individual's progress. Continuous monitoring might involve the use of wearable devices, such as accelerometers or heart rate monitors, that track performance in real-time. This data can be integrated with the results of periodic re-evaluations to provide a comprehensive picture of an individual's progress.

Integrating Evaluation into Training Programs

Tailoring Workloads Based on Evaluation Data

One of the key benefits of FEMD evaluation is the ability to tailor training workloads based on the data. This ensures that training is both effective and safe, helping to prevent overtraining and injuries.

- **Practical Examples of Data-Driven Training Adjustments**: If an evaluation shows that an athlete's bilateral balance is off, the training program might be adjusted to include more exercises that target the weaker side. Similarly, if the data shows a decline in velocity over multiple sets, the volume of training might be reduced to prevent fatigue.
- **Case Studies: Before and After Evaluation-Based Training**: Case studies can provide valuable insights into the effectiveness of evaluation-based training. They should highlight improvements in performance, strength, and other metrics that were achieved as a result of data-driven training adjustments.

Optimizing Progressions with FEMDs

Progressive overload is a key principle of training, but it must be carefully managed to avoid overtraining and injury. FEMD provides the data needed to optimize progressions and ensure that they are appropriate for the individual.

- **The Science of Progressive Overload in FEMD Context**: Progressive overload involves gradually increasing the demands placed on the body to stimulate adaptations such as increased strength, endurance, or power. FEMDs can be used to monitor how the body is responding to these increases in demand and to adjust the progression accordingly.
- **Strategies for Avoiding Overtraining**: Overtraining occurs when the volume and intensity of training exceed the body's ability to recover. This can lead to decreased performance, increased risk of injury, and other negative outcomes. FEMDs can help to prevent overtraining by providing data on fatigue, recovery, and other factors that affect performance.

Injury Prevention Through Evaluation

Injury prevention is a key goal of any training program, and FEMD evaluation can play a crucial role in identifying and addressing risk factors before they lead to injury.

- **Identifying Early Warning Signs with FEMD Metrics**: FEMDs can detect subtle changes in performance that may indicate the early stages of an injury. For example, a decline in bilateral balance or an increase in asymmetry between agonist and antagonist muscle groups can be early warning signs of an impending injury.
- **Designing Prehabilitative Programs Based on Evaluation Data**: Prehabilitation refers to the practice of using preventive exercises to strengthen areas of weakness and reduce the risk of injury. FEMD data can be used to design prehabilitative programs that target specific risk factors identified during an evaluation.

Feedback Loops and Real-Time Adaptations

One of the most powerful features of FEMD is its ability to provide real-time feedback, allowing for immediate adjustments during training.

- **The Role of Real-Time Feedback in Dynamic Training Environments**: Real-time feedback enhances the effectiveness of training by providing immediate information on performance. For example, if an athlete's velocity begins to drop during a set, the coach can intervene to adjust the load or technique.
- **Case Studies of Real-Time Adjustments and Their Outcomes**: For example, case studies show how athletes are able to improve their performance by making real-time adjustments based on FEMD feedback and its impact on training outcomes.

Conclusion

Summary of Key Points

This chapter has explored the various aspects of evaluation and measurement with functional electromechanical devices, including the proven validity and reliability of the technology, key metrics FEMDs can measure, evaluation protocols, and the integration of data into training programs.

Final Thoughts on the Future of Evaluation

As FEMD technology continues to evolve, it is likely to play an increasingly important role in the evaluation and optimization of physical performance. The ability to collect accurate, real-time data on a wide range of metrics provides valuable insights that can be used to enhance training, prevent injuries, and improve overall physical health. As researchers and practitioners continue to explore the possibilities of FEMD, the future of physical evaluation and training looks bright.

References

Andrades-Ramírez, Oscar, David Ulloa-Díaz, Bryan Alfaro Castillo, Patricio Arroyo-Jofré, Antonio Castillo-Paredes, and Luis Chirosa-Ríos. 2024. "Test—Retest Reliability of an Isometric and Isometric/Vibratory Muscular Strength Protocol with Functional Electro-Mechanical Dynamometry." *Sports* 12 (7): 175. Multidisciplinary Digital Publishing Institute. doi:10.3390/SPORTS12070175.

Baena-Raya, Andrés, David M. Díez-Fernández, Amador García-Ramos, Alberto Soriano-Maldonado, and Manuel A. Rodríguez-Pérez. 2021. "Concurrent Validity and Reliability of a Functional Electromechanical Dynamometer to Assess Isometric Mid-Thigh Pull Performance." *Proceedings of the Institution of Mechanical Engineers, Part P: Journal of Sports Engineering and Technology* 237 (3): 197–204. London, England: Sage. doi:10.1177/17543371211030180.

Chirosa-Ríos, Ignacio, Lorenzo Ruiz-Orellana, Luis Chirosa-Ríos, Indya Del-Cuerpo, Isidoro Martínez-Martín, Ángela Rodríguez-Perea, Ignacio Pelayo-Tejo, Daniel Jerez-Mayorga, and Darío Martinez-Garcia. 2022. "Defensive Two-Step Test in Handball Players: Reliability of a New Test for Assessing Displacement Velocity." *E-Balonmano* 18 (3): 233–244.

del Corral, Tamara, Álvaro Gómez Sánchez, and Ibai López-de-Uralde-Villanueva. 2020. "Test-Retest Reliability, Minimal Detectable Change and Minimal Clinically Important Differences in Modified Shuttle Walk Test in Children and Adolescents with Cystic Fibrosis." *Journal of Cystic Fibrosis* 19 (3): 442–448. Elsevier. doi:10.1016/J.JCF.2019.10.007.

del-Cuerpo, Indya, Daniel Jerez-Mayorga, Pedro Delgado-Floody, María Dolores Morenas-Aguilar, and Luis Javier Chirosa-Ríos. 2023. "Test-Retest Reliability of the Functional Electromechanical Dynamometer for Squat Exercise." *International Journal of Environmental Research and Public Health* 20 (2). doi:10.3390/IJERPH20021289.

García-Buendía, Gustavo, Ángela Rodríguez-Perea, Ignacio Chirosa-Ríos, Luis Javier Chirosa-Ríos, and Darío Martínez-García. 2024. "Reliability of Dynamic Shoulder Strength Test Battery Using Multi-Joint Isokinetic Device." *Sensors* 24 (11): 3568. Multidisciplinary Digital Publishing Institute. doi:10.3390/S24113568.

Hernández Sampieri, Roberto, Carlos Fernández Collado, and María del Pilar Baptista Lucio. 2014. *Metodología de La Investigación*. Mexico. www.uca.ac.cr/wp-content/uploads/2017/10/Investigacion.pdf.

Hopkins, W. 2000. "Measures of Reliability in Sports Medicine and Science." *Sports Medicine* 30 (1): 1–15. doi:10.2165/00007256-200030010-00001.

Hopkins, William G., Stephen W. Marshall, Alan M. Batterham, and Juri Hanin. 2009. "Progressive Statistics for Studies in Sports Medicine and

Exercise Science." *Medicine and Science in Sports and Exercise* 41 (1): 3–12. doi:10.1249/MSS.0b013e31818cb278.

Jerez-Mayorga, Daniel, Álvaro Huerta-Ojeda, Luis Javier Chirosa-Ríos, Francisco Guede-Rojas, Iris Paola Guzmán-Guzmán, Leonardo Intelangelo, Claudia Miranda-Fuentes, and Pedro Delgado-Floody. 2021. "Test—Retest Reliability of Functional Electromechanical Dynamometer on Five Sit-to-Stand Measures in Healthy Young Adults." *International Journal of Environmental Research and Public Health* 18 (13). MDPI AG. doi:10.3390/ijerph18136829.

Lawshe, C. H. 1975. "A Quantitative Approach to Content Validity." *Personnel Psychology* 28 (4): 563–575. John Wiley & Sons, Ltd. doi:10.1111/J.1744-6570.1975.TB01393.X.

Martin Bland, J., and Douglas G. Altman. 1986. "Statistical Methods for Assessing Agreement Between Two Methods of Clinical Measurement." *The Lancet* 327 (8476): 307–310. doi:10.1016/S0140-6736(86)90837-8.

Martin Bland, J., and Douglas G. Altman. 1995. "Comparing Methods of Measurement: Why Plotting Difference against Standard Method Is Misleading." *The Lancet* 346: 1085–1087. doi:10.1016/S0140-6736(95)91748-9.

Martinez-Garcia, Dario, Angela Rodriguez-Perea, Paola Barboza, David Ulloa-Díaz, Daniel Jerez-Mayorga, Ignacio Chirosa, and Luis Javier Chirosa Ríos. 2020. "Reliability of a Standing Isokinetic Shoulder Rotators Strength Test Using a Functional Electromechanical Dynamometer: Effects of Velocity." *PeerJ* 8 (October). PeerJ Inc. doi:10.7717/PEERJ.9951/SUPP-2.

McGuigan, Mike. 2020. *Testing and Evaluation of Strength and Power*. 1st Edition. Routledge.

Morenas-Aguilar, Maria Dolores, Luis J. Chirosa Rios, Angela Rodriguez-Perea, Juan Antonio Vázquez Diz, Ignacio J. Chirosa Rios, José Fernando Vera Vera, Lorenzo Ruiz-Orellana, and Daniel Jerez-Mayorga. 2023. "Test—Retest Reliability of 3 Specific Strength Tests in Professional Handball Players." *Journal of Sport Rehabilitation* 1 (aop): 1–10. Human Kinetics. doi:10.1123/JSR.2022-0267.

Reyes-Ferrada, Waleska, L. Chirosa-Rios, I. Chirosa-Rios, D. Martínez-Garcia, Paola Barboza-Gonzalez, D. Ulloa-Diaz, Daniel Jerez-Mayorga, and A. Rodríguez-Perea. 2022. "A New Reliable Device to Assess Trunk Extensors Strength." *Acta of Bioengineering and Biomechanics* 24 (1): 2022. doi:10.37190/ABB-01965-2021-05.

Rodriguez-Perea, Angela, L. J. Chirosa-Ríos, Dario Martinez-Garcia, David Ulloa-Díaz, Francisco Guede Rojas, Daniel Jerez-Mayorga, and Ignacio J. Chirosa Rios. 2019. "Reliability of Isometric and Isokinetic Trunk Flexor Strength Using a Functional Electromechanical Dynamometer." *PeerJ* 7 (10). doi:10.7717/peerj.7883.

Rodriguez-Perea, Ángela, D. Jerez-Mayorga, Amador García-Ramos, Dario Martínez-García, and Luis Javier Chirosa Ríos. 2021. "Reliability and Concurrent Validity of a Functional Electromechanical Dynamometer Device for the Assessment of Movement Velocity." *Proceedings of the Institution of Mechanical Engineers, Part P: Journal of Sports Engineering and Technology* 235 (January): 176–181. London, England: Sage. doi:10.1177/1754337120984883.

Rodríguez-Perea, Angela, M. D. Morenas Aguilar, Raquel Escobar-Molina, Darío Martínez-García, Ignacio Chirosa Ríos, Daniel Jerez-Mayorga, Luis Chirosa-Ríos, Danica Janicijevic, and Waleska Reyes-Ferrada. 2023. "Strength Assessment of Trunk Rotator Muscles: A Multicenter Reliability Study." *Healthcare* 11 (16): 2331. Multidisciplinary Digital Publishing Institute. doi:10.3390/HEALTHCARE11162331.

Sánchez-Sánchez, Antonio Jesús, Luis Javier Chirosa-Ríos, Ignacio Jesús Chirosa-Ríos, Agustín José García-Vega, and Daniel Jerez-Mayorga. 2021. "Test-Retest Reliability of a Functional Electromechanical Dynamometer on Swing Eccentric Hamstring Exercise Measures in Soccer Players." *PeerJ* 9 (July): e11743. PeerJ Inc. doi:10.7717/PEERJ.11743/SUPP-2.

Vega, Enrique Cerda, Daniel Jerez-Mayorga, Ramón Machado Payer, Christian Campos Jara, Iris Guzman-Guzman, Alvaro Reyes Ponce, and Luis Javier Chirosa. 2018. "Validity and Reliability of Evaluating Hip Abductor Strength Using Different Normalization Methods in a Functional Electromechanical Device." *PLoS One* 13 (8). doi:10.1371/JOURNAL.PONE.0202248.

Weir, Joseph P. 2005. "Quantifying Test-Retest Reliability Using the Intraclass Correlation Coefficient and the SEM." *Journal of Strength and Conditioning Research* 19 (1): 231–240. doi:10.1519/15184.1.

4 Methodology of Training with Functional Electromechanical Dynamometers

Ignacio J. Chirosa Rios

Introduction

Functional electromechanical dynamometers (FEMD) offer distinct advantages over other types of training devices. These include precise measurement and controlled resistance (Harris et al., 2022). Training methodologies using these devices can optimize training and enhance the effectiveness of training protocols for a diverse range of individuals—from elite athletes seeking to maximize their performance to individuals in rehabilitation working to restore functional capacity (Wilk et al., 2021). This chapter highlights how FEMDs can be employed to adapt exercises more effectively, ensuring that an individual's specific needs and goals are met with greater accuracy and efficiency. By integrating the detailed feedback and control provided by FEMD, traditional training approaches can be refined, introducing new methodologies that capitalize on the precision and adaptability of this advanced technology. Whether the goal is to improve physical fitness, enhance athletic performance, protect, prevent injuries, or support recovery from injury, the methodology discussed in this chapter offers innovative strategies for achieving optimal outcomes.

Through a comprehensive examination of these methodologies, practitioners, scientists, coaches, and therapists will gain and understand the tools and insights necessary to implement the FEMD in their practice effectively. This approach not only highlights the technological advantages of FEMD but also emphasizes the importance of individualized training, moving toward personalized "medicine" with the value of strength training, making it a valuable resource for anyone involved in the pursuit of physical improvement.

Before delving deeply into the intricacies of training with FEMD, it is essential to establish a foundation of precision. The ability to accurately select the specific expression of force to develop, and accurately position the stimulus on the force-velocity curve (FVC), is paramount to achieving optimal results (Jones et al., 2021). This is crucial and necessary; thus, one must be guided through the process of refining focus on the desired force expression—whether it be maximal strength, explosive power, or speed—and learn how to align training stimuli within the appropriate zones of the FVC (Santos & Silva, 2022).

DOI: 10.4324/9781003425182-5

As previously noted, the FVC is a fundamental tool in understanding how different types of strength and velocity interact within the body (Gonzalez-Badillo & Sanchez-Medina, 2010). By identifying the correct intervention zone on this curve, a practitioner can arrange training methods to target specific physiological adaptations. For instance, training in the high-force, low-velocity end of the curve will primarily enhance maximal strength, while focusing on the low-force, high-velocity end will develop speed and power (Cormie et al., 2011). This is a quick and easy explanation but knowing exactly what the target is makes it more likely that it will be reached.

As the chapter proceeds, it will explore the principles and applications that will enable a coach to construct a precise and personalized training program, supported by sports science and adjusted to the most important variables to design advanced strength training plans (Haff & Triplett, 2015).

There is a crucial aspect to designing effective and advanced training programs, which involves creating tasks or exercises that align with the specific focus required by the chosen method, through the correct selection of the expression of force. However, this is not the book that will provide specific tasks or exercises. Each sport, each discipline, and each professional should know how to design these tasks themselves. There is abundant literature available on this topic. In this manuscript, the goal is solely to guide coaches in the creation of the method (stimulus), so that it can be applied to the tasks that each sports science professional deems most appropriate (Bompa & Haff, 2009).

Training Perspectives: Functional versus Structural Approaches

Functional Training

Functional training is designed to enhance performance in specific movements or activities by improving neuromuscular coordination, balance, and overall movement efficiency. Unlike traditional strength training, which often focuses on isolating individual muscles, functional training emphasizes exercises that replicate the complex, multi-joint movements used in daily life and athletic activities. This type of training aims to develop sport-specific abilities by targeting the muscle groups and movement patterns that are most relevant to an athlete's sport or activity.

For instance, a basketball player might engage in functional training that includes plyometric exercises to improve their explosive power for jumping, or agility drills to enhance their ability to change direction quickly. Similarly, a swimmer might focus on exercises that improve their core stability and shoulder mobility, which are crucial for effective stroke technique. By focusing on the specific demands of a sport, functional training helps athletes not only improve their performance but also reduce the risk of injury by strengthening the muscles and joints in a way that directly translates to their sport.

Additionally, functional training is beneficial for non-athletes as well. For those looking to improve their overall fitness or ability to perform daily tasks, functional exercises like squats, lunges, and rotational movements can enhance strength, flexibility, and coordination in a way that supports everyday activities. Ultimately, functional training is about creating a stronger, more adaptable body that is capable of performing a wide range of movements with efficiency and ease, whether on the field of play or in daily life.

Structural Training

Increasing muscle mass, known as hypertrophy, and enhancing maximal strength are fundamental goals in many strength training programs. These goals are achieved by focusing on the recruitment and growth of muscle fibers through targeted resistance training. This type of training is essential for athletes who are looking to build a solid foundation of strength that can be further developed for sport-specific purposes. For athletes, hypertrophy training serves as a preparatory phase that builds the necessary muscle size and strength to support more advanced, sport-specific training. This propaedeutic approach ensures that athletes have the muscular capacity to handle the demands of their sport, whether it involves explosive power, endurance, or agility.

On the other hand, hypertrophy and strength training extend far beyond athletic performance and serve a wide array of purposes for different populations. For individuals focused on health, this type of training is crucial for maintaining or improving muscle mass, which is essential for metabolic health, bone density, and overall physical function. As people age, maintaining muscle mass becomes increasingly important to prevent sarcopenia, reduce the risk of falls, and maintain independence.

For those interested in aesthetics, hypertrophy training is often the primary focus. This type of training emphasizes the development of muscle size and definition, leading to the muscular physique often associated with bodybuilding. It's a versatile approach that can be tailored to individual goals, whether one is aiming to build a lean, toned body or achieve a more muscular, bulked-up appearance.

Moreover, for those engaging in strength training for leisure or personal fulfillment, the benefits are multifaceted. Beyond the physical improvements, training for hypertrophy can enhance mental well-being, boost confidence, and provide a sense of accomplishment. Whether the goal is to enhance athletic performance, improve health, achieve aesthetic goals, or simply enjoy the process of getting stronger, hypertrophy and maximal strength training offer a comprehensive approach that can be adapted to meet diverse needs and objectives.

Functional versus Structural: Which Approach Is Right?

One of the initial steps in the process of determining a training program is to select the most suitable training approach, personalized to the specific goals and needs of the individual or group in question. This decision is foundational, as it will guide the entire training program and influence every aspect of its design, from the selection of exercises and the structure of workouts to the progression of intensity and the overall timeline.

Choosing the right training approach requires careful consideration of various factors, including the athlete's current fitness level, previous training experience, the specific objectives they aim to achieve, and any unique physical or psychological characteristics they may have. For instance, an athlete preparing for a competition might require a highly specific and periodized approach that prioritizes performance outcomes, while someone seeking general fitness or rehabilitation might benefit more from a balanced, holistic program that incorporates elements of strength, flexibility, and endurance.

This step is also critical in aligning the training program with the available resources, such as equipment, time, and support systems, ensuring that the approach is not only effective but also practical and sustainable. By carefully selecting the most appropriate training approach, the stage is set for a targeted and efficient program that maximizes the potential for success and minimizes the risk of injury or burnout.

Functional methods (see Figure 4.1) aim to improve strength from a functional point of view, that is, each Newton (N) of force that is gained should be

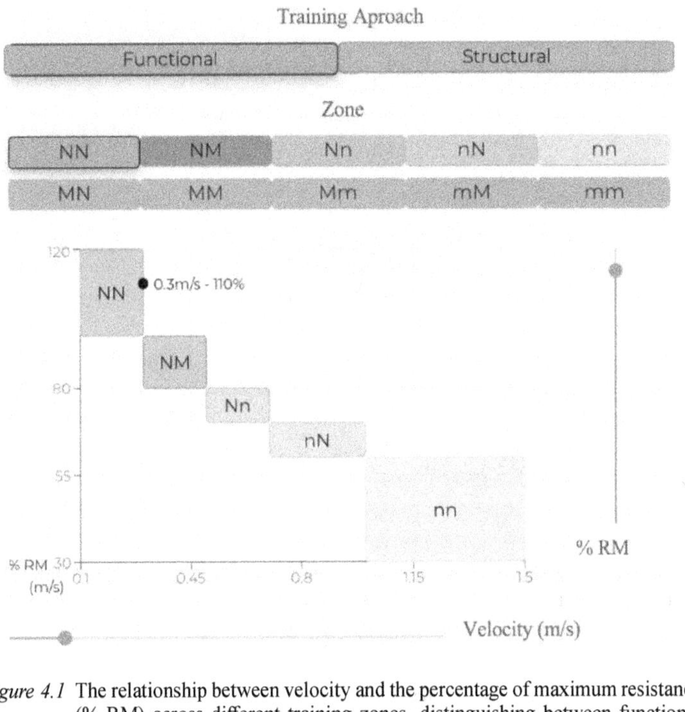

Figure 4.1 The relationship between velocity and the percentage of maximum resistance (% RM) across different training zones, distinguishing between functional and structural approaches. It highlights how various force expression zones align with specific velocities and load intensities, guiding the selection of training protocols to target functional performance.

focused on improving the activity being performed or a specific task performance, whether it is high-level sport or activities of daily life. That force must be applied to the gesture or skill to be improved. For example, an increase in strength in the knee extensor musculature would improve gestures such as jumping or increase movement velocity. The velocity of displacement or muscle tension should be the maximum possible. The time to reach the maximum value should be as short as possible.

However, the final objective of *Structural methods* (see Figure 4.2) is to improve the cross section area (CSA) of the muscle, or in other words, to promote hypertrophy as an adaptive response. In all of these methods, the execution speed is not the maximum possible. It is compromised in favor of the metabolic and mechanical mechanisms that are provoked in the set of fibers involved. There are three mechanisms by which hypertrophy is induced (Schoenfeld, 2012). These three mechanisms—mechanical tension, muscle

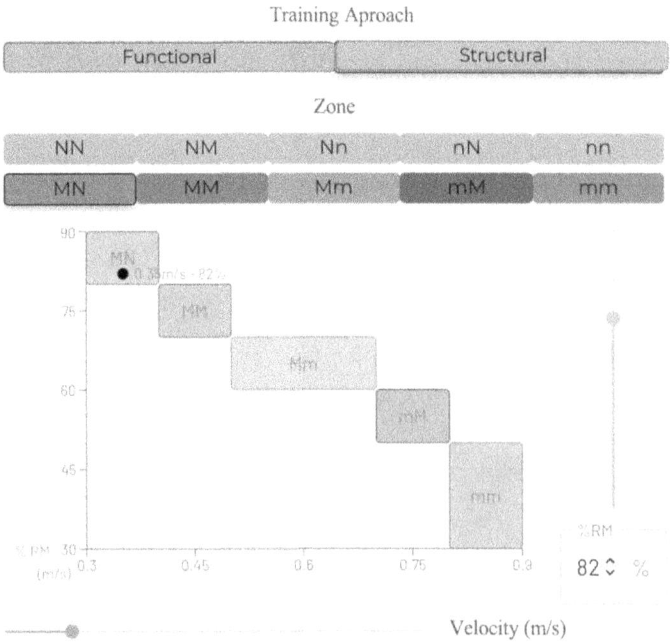

Figure 4.2 The relationship between velocity and the percentage of maximum resistance (% RM) within the context of different training zones, highlighting both functional and structural approaches. The graph displays how various zones correlate with specific velocities and load intensities. This visualization aids in selecting appropriate training protocols to target structural development searching for increasing muscle mass.

damage, and metabolic stress—work synergistically to induce muscle hypertrophy, with each playing a unique role in the growth and adaptation of muscle tissue in response to resistance training. At least two of them must be stimulated in order to provoke the creation of muscle mass and thus an increase in CSA, regardless of the type of fiber (IIx, IIa, I), including connective structures (Schoenfeld, 2013).

Zones to Improve Different Expressions of Force

In strength training, different zones can be targeted to improve specific expressions of force. Each zone employs specific load percentages, velocities, and training focuses to achieve desired adaptations. Here's a detailed breakdown:

Zone 10. Neural-Neural (NN)

Focus: Maximum Strength and Recruitment
Concentric Load: 90%–100% of 1RM (MDFc)
Eccentric Load: 110%–120% of 1RM (MDFc)
Execution Velocity: Below 0.3 m/s for concentric and 0.4 m/s for eccentric actions
Objective: Maximize muscle tension and recruitment at both spatial and temporal levels.

These methods involve the use of high external resistance and very slow execution speeds, typically below 0.3 m/s, or 0.4 m/s in the case of pure eccentric actions. The key criterion is the achievement of maximum muscular tension, with both spatial and temporal recruitment reaching their peak levels. Intervention in this zone can be accomplished through dynamic loads, whether concentric or eccentric, as well as through maximal isometrics, either in isolation or combined with dynamic movements. The term "NN" signifies that these are purely neural methods, focused on optimizing the nervous system's ability to generate and sustain high levels of force.

Zone 9. Neural-Morphological (NM)

Focus: Selective Hypertrophy with High Neural Component
Load: 80%–95% of 1RM (MDFc)
Time Under Tension (TUT): Increased, reaching muscle failure is acceptable with complete recovery.
Execution Velocity: Small or non-existent velocity reserve.
Objective: Stimulate neural adaptations and selective hypertrophy (IIx, mainly) depending on the athlete's functional profile.

This zone of intervention is a little lower than the NN. This set of methods uses high external resistance magnitudes, medium-low execution speed, between 0.3 m/s and 0.7 m/s. The determining factor is that there is maximum muscular tension and that recruitment, both spatially and temporally, is at a maximum. By increasing the TUT, not only neural adaptations are produced but also structural adaptations of the set of fibers associated with IIx and IIb. In compound methods, these loads are suitable to form the *heavy part of the contrasts*. As the load percentage is lowered, approaching 80%, it is necessary to consider the inclusion of some repetitions in reserve (RIR).

Zone 8. Neural-Neural (Nn): Power Development Focus with high loads

Focus: Dynamic Efforts and Intermuscular Coordination
Load: 70%–80% of 1RM
Execution Velocity: 0.5–0.7 m/s
Objective: Improve intermuscular coordination and segmental speed.

"Nn" refers to the zone where maximum power output should be achieved. In this zone, the external load or resistance is substantial enough to enable the expression of maximum power. The focus is on optimizing intermuscular coordination using significant loads, typically ranging between 70% and 80% of MDF. When considering velocity, this corresponds to a spectrum of 0.5 to 0.7 m/s. Compound movements can still be effectively performed within this range, making these loads ideal for the "heavy" component of contrast training. At this stage, it becomes crucial to determine the desired repetition reserve (RIR) to balance power output with endurance and recovery.

Zone 7. Neural-Neural (nN): Power Development Focus with Lower Loads

Focus: Execution Speed and Power
Load: 60%–70% of 1RM
Execution Speed: 0.7–1 m/s
Objective: Enhance segmental speed and maintain intermuscular coordination with minimal speed loss (10%–15%).

"nN" represents a zone still dedicated to power development but with a distinct emphasis on the speed of execution. The primary goal here is to enhance segmental speed, which is crucial for optimizing the efficiency and effectiveness of movement patterns. Intermuscular coordination becomes paramount in this zone, as it is essential to ensure that the muscle chains involved in specific gestures or actions are seamlessly integrated and function in harmony.

A key factor in this zone is managing the RIR, which are critical for maintaining the intended speed of the movement. Attention must be paid to avoid fatigue that could compromise velocity; therefore, the number of sets and repetitions should be carefully controlled to prevent excessive prolongation. Additionally, it is vital to monitor the loss of speed during exercises, which should be limited to no more than 10%–15% to ensure that the training remains focused on developing speed and not endurance or strength. This approach ensures that the power output remains high and that the athlete can effectively translate this power into quick, explosive actions in their specific sport or activity.

Zone 6. Neural-Neural (nn)

Focus: Segmental Speed Improvement
Load: 30%–60% of 1RM
Execution Velocity: 1–1.5 m/s
Objective: Improve velocity without significant strength gains, focusing on intermuscular coordination and reactive actions.

As in the "nN" zone, intermuscular coordination is crucial. The seamless integration of the muscle chains involved in the specific gestures or movements being trained is essential for maximizing velocity. Proper coordination allows for the rapid execution of movements with minimal loss of force, ensuring that the athlete can perform at their highest possible speed.

Managing repetitions in reserve (RIR) is a critical aspect of training in the "nn" zone. The goal is to maintain the speed of execution throughout the set, avoiding fatigue that could slow down the movement and detract from the desired training outcome. The number of repetitions should be carefully controlled, and the sets should not be extended to the point where speed significantly declines.

Depending on the period of the season and the athlete's overall training phase, the acceptable loss of speed during exercises can vary. In some cases, a speed loss of 10%–15% might be acceptable, allowing for a balance between maintaining speed and achieving some degree of muscular fatigue. However, in other scenarios, particularly when the focus is solely on speed development, a greater tolerance of 20%–30% speed loss may be permitted, especially if the athlete is transitioning from a strength-focused phase and needs to recalibrate their neuromuscular system for speed. This flexibility ensures that training remains adaptable to the athlete's needs while still prioritizing the development of segmental velocity.

Zone 5. Morphological-Neural (MN)

Focus: Borderline Neural and Hypertrophy Adaptations
Load: 70%–85% of 1RM

Execution Velocity: 0.4–0.7 m/s (values as a reference; velocity here does not matter)
Repetitions: Five to eight, with one to two repetitions in reserve (RIRs) for power focus.
Objective: Maximize hypertrophy while maintaining high work speeds.

This set of methods is particularly effective for inducing hypertrophy, targeting the growth of muscle mass through specific training protocols. Typically, the repetition range for these exercises falls between five and eight reps, a sweet spot that balances intensity and volume to stimulate muscle growth. The velocity during these movements generally ranges from 0.4 to 0.7 m/s. However, because these are structural methods focused on maximizing hypertrophy, it may be beneficial to further reduce the speed to enhance the time under tension, thereby optimizing the mechanical stress placed on the muscles.

The number of sets can vary significantly depending on several factors, including the training phase within the season, the specific goals of the selected program, and the athlete's current level of fitness. In the early stages of a training cycle or for athletes with a higher tolerance for volume, the number of sets might range from 8 to 12 or even exceed 12 sets per muscle group in a single session. If the training focus shifts toward power development within a hypertrophy-oriented program, it is crucial to manage fatigue effectively. In such cases, it is advisable to leave one or two RIR at the end of each set. This approach ensures that the athlete maintains high movement quality and explosive intent, avoiding excessive fatigue that could diminish the effectiveness of the power development. Balancing the volume, intensity, and velocity of these methods is key to achieving the desired hypertrophic and performance outcomes, allowing for a versatile and adaptable training regimen that meets the evolving needs of the athlete.

Zone 4. Morphological-Morphological (MM)

Focus: General Hypertrophy
Load: 70%–80% of 1RM
Execution Velocity: Controlled, with low RIR (10/12).
Objective: Increase muscle cross-sectional area through high mechanical and metabolic stress.

The load range of 70%–80% of maximum capacity is widely recognized as the most representative for hypertrophy-focused training methods. This range has traditionally been the foundation for bodybuilding techniques, commonly referred to as multiple repetition methods. These methods are specifically designed to generate high levels of metabolic stress while simultaneously maintaining a load significant enough to induce optimal mechanical stress on the muscles.

This combination of metabolic and mechanical stress is essential for eliciting the physiological responses necessary for hypertrophy. By working within this load range, the muscles are subjected to conditions that favor the synthesis of new muscle proteins, leading to increased muscle mass over time. The dual approach of applying substantial resistance while driving metabolic fatigue ensures that the muscles are adequately challenged, promoting growth through both structural adaptation and increased endurance.

Furthermore, these methods are not only effective for general hypertrophic responses but also adaptable to different training phases and individual needs. By carefully adjusting variables such as the number of repetitions, sets, and rest periods, this approach can be tailored to achieve specific hypertrophy goals, whether it be for aesthetic purposes, sport-specific strength, or overall muscular development. The strategic use of this load range, combined with proper training progression, forms a robust framework for achieving significant and sustained muscle growth.

Zone 3. Morphological-Morphological (Mm)

Focus: Specific Hypertrophy
Load: 60%–70% of 1RM
Execution Velocity: Sub-maximal or slow.
Objective: Tissue adaptation and preliminary work for maximal loads.

These load ranges are particularly well-suited for inducing hypertrophy, especially in individuals who have already developed a foundational level of experience in resistance training. At the lower end of the spectrum, working with 60% of the MDF provides the minimum mechanical stimulus necessary to elicit hypertrophic responses. This level is ideal for those transitioning from beginner to intermediate training stages, as it effectively introduces the muscle to the necessary stress required for growth without overwhelming the neuromuscular system.

For those with an intermediate to advanced training background, increasing the load to around 70% of the MDF is recommended to further stimulate muscle hypertrophy. At this stage, the use of more sophisticated techniques, such as supersets, drop sets, or strategies involving pre- or post-exhaustion, can significantly enhance the hypertrophic effect. These methods not only increase the total time under tension but also maximize the recruitment of muscle fibers, leading to more comprehensive muscle development.

Furthermore, these load ranges are particularly effective for creating metabolic adaptations, as they strike an optimal balance between mechanical stress and metabolic demand. The combination of moderate to high resistance with increased metabolic stress fosters an environment highly conducive to muscle growth. This approach not only promotes the synthesis of new muscle proteins but also enhances muscle endurance, allowing for sustained improvements over time. By carefully managing these loads within a well-structured training program, individuals can achieve significant gains in muscle size and overall strength, making this approach a cornerstone of effective hypertrophy training.

Zone 2. Morphological-Morphological (mM)

Focus: Strength Endurance and Structural Adaptations
Load: 50%–60% of 1RM
Execution Velocity: Controlled.
Objective: Enhance strength endurance and post-match recovery, or structural improvement for advanced athletes.

This intervention zone is often employed when working with beginners, typically following an initial phase where the focus has been on learning and mastering the correct techniques for basic strength training movements. At this stage, the primary objective is to establish a solid foundation of movement quality and muscular endurance, ensuring that the individual can perform exercises safely and effectively as they progress to more challenging loads.

For more advanced athletes, this load range becomes particularly valuable in the development of strength endurance, making it ideally suited for those involved in long-duration cyclic sports, such as cycling, rowing, or running. In these sports, the ability to sustain muscular effort over extended periods is crucial. By focusing on moderate loads, athletes can build the muscular stamina necessary to maintain high levels of performance throughout prolonged activities. This approach not only enhances endurance but also reinforces proper movement patterns, which is essential for preventing fatigue-related injuries that can occur during repetitive, long-duration events.

Moreover, this load range allows for a balanced approach that combines strength and endurance training. By carefully managing the volume and intensity of the workouts, athletes can improve their ability to resist fatigue, maintain power output over time, and enhance overall athletic performance. This makes the intervention zone not just a bridge for beginners, but also a critical component of advanced training programs aimed at optimizing endurance and durability in competitive environments.

Zone 1. Morphological-Morphological (mm)

Focus: Initial Adaptations for Beginners
Load: Less than 50% of 1RM
Execution Velocity: Slow, with high repetitions.
Objective: Induce initial hypertrophy responses and adaptation in novices, suitable for recovery and protection tasks.

This range represents the lowest zone for the development of general hypertrophy. These percentages are commonly applied in the initial stages of strength training, particularly for those new to the basic movements and for eliciting early adaptation responses in individuals with no prior experience in external resistance training.

When paired with occlusive training strategies, these lower load percentages can effectively induce significant metabolic effects, triggering hypertrophic mechanisms. However, on their own, these percentages are relatively low and require a high number of repetitions to elicit any substantial structural adaptation. As a result, they are primarily suited for early-stage training or foundational work before progressing to higher intensities.

Figure 4.3 illustrates the background for understanding the balance required in training stimulus to elicit specific adaptation responses. In the context of this book, these methodologies integrate new technology such as functional electromechanical dynamometers. The diagram illustrates three critical zones: Neutral Stimulus, Optimum Stimulus, and Excessive Stimulus or Over-Stimulation, each with distinct impacts on training outcomes (see Figure 4.3).

In the Neutral Stimulus zone, the applied load or intensity does not meet the minimum adaptation threshold, resulting in negligible physiological or performance improvements. This highlights the importance of appropriately calibrating training loads to avoid ineffective training sessions. On the opposite end, the Excessive Stimulus or Over-Stimulation zone indicates that the applied stimulus—whether in terms of intensity or volume—is too high, leading to potential

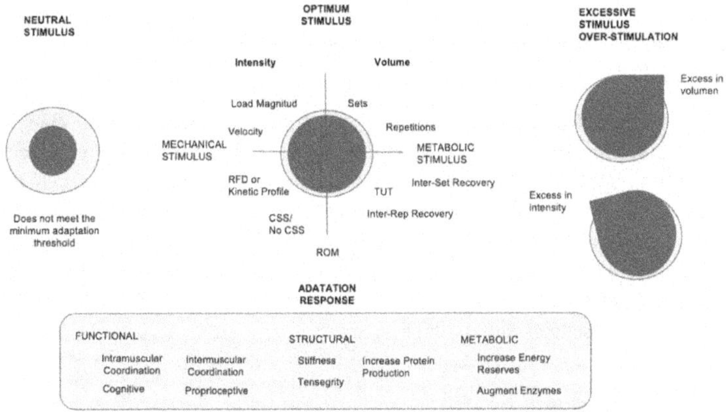

Figure 4.3 The relationship between training stimuli and their adaptive responses, highlighting three key zones: Neutral Stimulus, Stimulus Optimum, and Excessive Stimulus/Over-Stimulation. It shows how appropriate mechanical and metabolic stimuli, when balanced in intensity and volume, can drive functional, structural, and metabolic adaptations. It emphasizes the need to stay within the optimal stimulus range to avoid insufficient adaptation or over-stimulation, which could lead to negative effects.

overtraining, injury, or maladaptation. Such over-stimulation can result in excessive volume or intensity that overwhelms the body's adaptive capacity, stressing the importance of careful monitoring and adjustment of training loads.

The core of effective training lies within the Optimum Stimulus zone, where both mechanical and metabolic stimuli are balanced to produce the desired adaptation responses. This zone is characterized by the correct combination of intensity (including load magnitude, velocity, and Rate of Force Development or RFD) and volume (such as sets, repetitions, and time under tension). The diagram underscores the significance of maintaining this balance to ensure that training is both challenging and productive, without tipping into undertraining or overtraining (see Figure 4.3).

Functional electromechanical dynamometers offer a precise tool for managing this balance by providing real-time feedback on key variables such as velocity, force, and power output. This technology allows for the fine-tuning of training protocols to maintain athletes within the Optimum Stimulus zone. By utilizing FEMD, coaches and practitioners can ensure that mechanical stimuli like load and velocity are precisely controlled, and metabolic demands are met without exceeding the athlete's capacity for adaptation. This integration of FEMD into training programs aligns with the diagram's emphasis on tailored, data-driven training approaches that optimize functional, structural, and metabolic adaptations. The precise monitoring capabilities of FEMD can also help in dynamically adjusting training loads and recovery times, thereby preventing the pitfalls of neutral or excessive stimuli and promoting sustained, progressive development of athletic performance.

Functional Electromechanical Devices and Their Operation

Functional electromechanical devices represent a class of advanced machinery that seamlessly integrates electrical, mechanical, and digital components to perform specific, often complex, functions (Rodriguez-Perea et al., 2019). These devices are at the forefront of modern automation and precision engineering, playing a critical role in industries such as robotics, manufacturing, healthcare, and more. The main purpose of FEMDs is to convert electrical energy into mechanical motion and, in some cases, to perform feedback control by integrating sensors and digital systems.

Basic Components of FEMD

FEMDs typically consist of several core components:

a. Power Supply: Provides the necessary electrical energy to the device. This can be in the form of direct current (DC) or alternating current (AC), depending on the device's design.

b. Actuators: These are the components that convert electrical energy into mechanical motion. Common types include electric motors, solenoids, and piezoelectric actuators.
c. Sensors: Sensors are used to monitor various parameters, such as position, force, temperature, and more. These provide feedback to the control system, allowing for precise operation and adjustments in real time.
d. Control System: This includes microcontrollers or digital signal processors (DSPs) that process input from sensors and command the actuators accordingly. The control system is the brain of the FEMDs, executing algorithms to perform the desired functions.
e. Mechanical Components: These include gears, levers, and other mechanical linkages that translate the actuator's motion into the required mechanical output.
f. Communication Interfaces: These allow the FEMDs to connect with other systems, such as computers, other devices, or networks, enabling data exchange and remote control.

How FEMDs Work

The operation of FEMDs can be understood through a step-by-step process:

1. Input Signal Reception: The device receives input signals from a user interface or an automated system. This could be a simple on/off command, a variable control signal, or data from a remote system.
2. Signal Processing: The control system interprets the input signal and, using pre-programmed algorithms, determines the appropriate response. This may involve processing data from sensors to ensure that the device's output meets the desired specifications.
3. Actuation: Based on the control system's instructions, actuators within the device convert electrical energy into mechanical motion. For example, an electric motor might rotate a shaft, or a solenoid might create a linear movement.
4. Feedback Loop: Sensors continuously monitor the device's operation, providing real-time data to the control system. This feedback is crucial for maintaining accuracy, especially in applications requiring high precision.
5. Output: The mechanical motion generated by the actuators is then used to perform the desired function. This could range from moving a robotic arm to compressing a material or even generating a vibration.
6. Communication and Data Storage: Many modern FEMDs are equipped with communication interfaces that allow them to send performance data to external systems for monitoring and analysis. This is essential for predictive maintenance and optimizing the operation of the device over time.

Modifying Resistance and Velocity with Electric Motors

One of the most innovative aspects of FEMDs is the ability to dynamically modify resistance or velocity during any phase of motion, whether in the concentric (muscle shortening) or eccentric (muscle lengthening) phases (Rodriguez-Perea et al., 2021). This capability is primarily achieved through the use of advanced electric motors that are controlled by sophisticated algorithms.

Electric Motors and Variable Resistance/Velocity

At the heart of this functionality are electric motors, which can precisely control the amount of force or speed applied during an exercise. These motors can adjust their torque output instantaneously, responding to real-time feedback from sensors that monitor the user's performance.

The resistance can be modified on the fly during any phase of movement. For example, the device can increase resistance during the eccentric phase to enhance muscle tension or decrease it during the concentric phase to allow for faster movement. This dynamic adjustment is crucial for creating specific training stimuli that are tailored to the user's needs.

Similarly, the speed at which the exercise is performed can be controlled with high precision. The device can slow down or speed up movements based on the desired training effect, such as improving muscle power or endurance.

Infinite Training Stimuli

By altering the load (force), velocity, and power output during any phase of an exercise, the possibilities for creating diverse training stimuli are virtually endless. This level of customization allows for targeted training that can improve specific physical attributes, such as strength, speed, or power, in a highly controlled manner.

The ability to fine-tune these variables opens *a new era of strength training*. The combinations of load, velocity, and power that can be applied during an exercise are almost infinite, offering unprecedented levels of precision in training (Chirosa-Ríos et al., 2022). This technology enables the design of highly specific training protocols that can cater to individual needs, whether for rehabilitation, athletic performance, or general fitness.

Uncharted Potential

Despite the clear potential, the full range of possibilities offered by these technologies remains largely unexplored. The fitness and sports science communities are only beginning to understand how these capabilities can be harnessed to optimize training outcomes. As more research is conducted, it is likely that new training methodologies and protocols will be developed, further revolutionizing the field of strength training (Torres-Banduc et al., 2023).

Real-Time Feedback and Adaptive Exercise

Another revolutionary aspect of FEMDs is the integration of real-time feedback systems. This technology significantly enhances the user experience and effectiveness of training (Andrades-Ramírez et al., 2024).

Sensors embedded in the device instantaneously and continuously collect data on various parameters, such as force, speed, and position. This data is processed and presented to the user in real-time, allowing them to adjust their performance on the spot.

With real-time feedback, users can make immediate adjustments to their technique, resistance, or speed during an exercise. For example, if the device detects that the user is struggling with a particular repetition, it can automatically reduce the resistance to ensure that the exercise is completed with proper form.

The ability to adapt exercises in real time makes each session more personalized and responsive to the user's current physical state. This leads to more effective workouts, as the training is always aligned with the user's capabilities at any given moment.

Real-time feedback also serves as a motivational tool. Users can see their performance metrics improving in real time, which can encourage them to push harder and achieve better results.

Classification of Different Stimuli

Given the advanced capabilities of FEMDs, it is possible to classify the various stimuli that can be generated during exercise. These can be broadly categorized into:

1. Strength Stimuli:
   Focus on maximizing muscle force output.
   Typically involves high resistance with controlled movement speeds.
2. Power Stimuli:
   Aims to improve explosive strength.
   Involves moderate to high resistance with high-speed movements.
3. Endurance Stimuli:
   Designed to enhance muscular endurance.
   Characterized by lower resistance with sustained, repetitive movements.
4. Hypertrophy Stimuli:
   Targets muscle growth by maximizing muscle tension over time.
   Involves moderate resistance with slower, controlled movements to increase time under tension.
5. Rehabilitation Stimuli:
   Focuses on gradual strength rebuilding and joint stabilization.
   Typically involves low resistance with highly controlled, slow movements.

6. Neuromuscular Efficiency Stimuli:
   Aims to improve the coordination between the nervous system and muscles. Often involves complex, multi-joint movements with varying resistance and speed.
7. Balance and Stability Stimuli:
   Enhances proprioception and the ability to maintain stability under varying conditions.

Often involve dynamic adjustments in resistance or movement direction to challenge the user's balance.

Functional electromechanical devices are transforming the landscape of strength training and rehabilitation. The ability to dynamically modify resistance and velocity during any phase of motion, coupled with real-time feedback, offers unparalleled opportunities to create personalized and highly effective training programs. As research into these technologies continues, the full potential of FEMDs will likely be uncovered, ushering in a new era of precision training that could redefine the approach to physical conditioning and rehabilitation. With infinite possibilities for training stimuli, FEMDs are set to become an indispensable tool in the quest for optimal performance and health.

Creating an Exercise with Functional Electromechanical Devices

Creating an exercise with a functional electromechanical device involves several steps, each designed to tailor the exercise to the specific needs and goals of the user. The process leverages the device's advanced capabilities to control resistance, velocity, and other variables dynamically throughout the exercise. Although various types of FEMDs are available on the market, the following section provides a basic guide on creating an exercise using an FEMD for illustrative purposes.

Step 1: Define the Exercise Goals

Before setting up the exercise on an FEMD, it's crucial to clearly define the goals. These goals will guide the selection of parameters and settings. Common goals include:

- **Strength Building**: Focus on increasing the amount of force that muscles can exert.
- **Power Development**: Aim to enhance explosive movements by combining force and speed.
- **Endurance Training**: Prolong muscle exertion over time to improve stamina.
- **Rehabilitation**: Gradually rebuild strength and mobility after an injury.
- **Hypertrophy**: Promote muscle growth through sustained tension.

Step 2: Select the Appropriate Mode

FEMDs offer various operational modes that provide different types of resistance and movement patterns. These include:

1. **Tonic Mode**: Ideal for simulating free weights with constant resistance.
2. **Kinetic Mode**: Best for controlling movement speed and direction, useful in rehabilitation and athletic training.
3. **Conic Mode**: Suited for functional training where resistance varies naturally with movement.
4. **Elastic Mode**: Mimics elastic bands with increasing resistance as the device is extended.
5. **Inertial Mode**: Perfect for power training, where resistance increases with speed.
6. **Isometric Mode**: Focuses on static strength by holding positions against resistance.
7. **Vibratory Mode**: Enhances muscle activation and circulation through added vibrations.

Step 3: Set the Exercise Parameters

Once the mode has been selected, specific parameters for the exercise can be set. These include:

- **Load (Force)**: Determine the amount of resistance to be applied. This can be adjusted based on the user's strength level and the specific phase of the exercise (concentric or eccentric).
- **Velocity**: Set the speed of movement for both the concentric and eccentric phases. This is particularly important in power and rehabilitation exercises.
- **Range of Motion**: Define the start and end points of the movement. In some modes, this can be dynamically adjusted based on real-time feedback.
- **Repetition and Set Configuration**: Decide the number of repetitions per set, the number of sets, and the rest time between sets.
- **Advanced Settings**: For more complex exercises, you might want to adjust additional settings like the frequency of data sampling, the activation of input/output triggers, and safety limits.

Step 4: Calibrate and Test the Exercise

Before beginning the full exercise routine, it's important to calibrate the device. This involves:

- **Calibration**: The FEMD will adjust to the initial position and ensure that all sensors and actuators are correctly aligned. The device may require the user to perform a few trial movements to establish baselines for force and velocity.

- **Testing**: Perform a few repetitions to ensure that the settings are appropriate and comfortable. This also allows the user to get a feel for the exercise and make any necessary adjustments before starting the full session.

Step 5: Execute the Exercise

With the device calibrated and the settings confirmed, the exercise can be executed. During the exercise:

- **Real-Time Feedback**: The FEMD provides real-time data on metrics such as force, speed, range of motion, and more. This feedback can be displayed on a monitor and used to adjust the exercise in real-time.
- **Adjustments**: Based on the feedback, the user or trainer can make immediate adjustments to resistance, speed, or even the exercise parameters to ensure optimal performance and safety.
- **Data Collection**: The device collects detailed data on each repetition, which can be analyzed to assess performance and make future training decisions.

Step 6: Review and Analyze the Exercise Data

After completing the exercise, the data collected by the FEMD can be reviewed. This includes:

- **Performance Metrics**: Analyze data such as peak force, average force, power output, and movement speed.
- **Progress Tracking**: Compare current data with previous sessions to track progress and make informed adjustments to future exercises.
- **Customization**: Use the insights gained from the data to customize future exercises, potentially altering resistance, velocity, or range of motion to better align with the user's evolving goals.

Step 7: Save and Share Exercise Data

Finally, the exercise data can be saved and shared:

- **Saving**: Store the data on an external drive, cloud service, or directly on the device for later analysis.
- **Sharing**: Send the data to a connected app or platform where it can be reviewed by a coach, therapist, or the user for further insights.

As technology continues to advance, the field of strength and conditioning is poised on the brink of significant breakthroughs. Innovations such as virtual reality training environments and advanced biomechanical simulations through motorized devices offer unprecedented opportunities to enhance athlete performance in controlled, risk-free settings. Additionally, the increasing trend toward personalized training programs—tailored to individual genetic profiles—promises a future where training efficiency is maximized, and injury risks are minimized (Joyner & Coyle, 2008).

References

Andrades-Ramírez, O., Ulloa-Díaz, D., Alfaro Castillo, B., Arroyo-Jofré, P., Castillo-Paredes, A., & Chirosa-Ríos, L. (2024). Test—retest reliability of an isometric and isometric/vibratory muscular strength protocol with functional electro-mechanical dynamometry. *Sports*, 12(7), 175.

Bompa, T. O., & Haff, G. G. (2009). *Periodization: Theory and methodology of training*. Human Kinetics.

Chirosa-Ríos, I. J., Ruiz Orellana, L., Chirosa-Ríos, L. J., Cuerpo, I. D., Martínez Martín, I., Rodríguez Perea, Á., Pelayo-Tejo, I., Jerez-Mayorga, D., & Martinez Garcia, D. (2022). Defensive two-step test in handball players: Reliability of a new test for assessing displacement velocity. *E-Balonmano*, 18(3), 233–244.

Cormie, P., McGuigan, M. R., & Newton, R. U. (2011). Developing maximal neuromuscular power: Part 1—biological basis of maximal power production. *Sports Medicine*, 41(1), 17–38.

Gonzalez-Badillo, J. J., & Sanchez-Medina, L. (2010). Movement velocity as a measure of loading intensity in resistance training. *International Journal of Sports Medicine*, 31(5), 347–352.

Haff, G. G., & Triplett, N. T. (2015). *Essentials of strength training and conditioning* (4th ed.). Human Kinetics.

Harris, N. K., Cronin, J. B., & Hopkins, W. G. (2022). Power outputs of a functional electromechanical dynamometer: Implications for functional exercise training. *Journal of Strength and Conditioning Research*, 36(1), 202–210.

Jones, P. A., Bampouras, T. M., & Marrin, K. (2021). An investigation into the force-velocity characteristics of isokinetic dynamometry and its implications for functional exercise. *Journal of Sports Sciences*, 39(5), 550–558.

Joyner, M. J., & Coyle, E. F. (2008). Endurance exercise performance: The physiology of champions. *The Journal of Physiology*, 586(1), 35–44. https://doi.org/10.1113/JPHYSIOL.2007.143834

Rodriguez-Perea, A., Jerez-Mayorga, D., García-Ramos, A, Martínez-García, D., & Chirosa-Ríos, L. J. (2021). Reliability and concurrent validity of a functional electromechanical dynamometer device for the assessment of movement velocity. *Proceedings of the Institution of Mechanical Engineers, Part P: Journal of Sports Engineering and Technology*, 235(3), 176–181. https://doi.org/10.1177/1754337120984883

Rodriguez-Perea, A., Chirosa-Ríos, L. J., Martinez-Garcia, D., Ulloa-Díaz, D., Guede Rojas, F., Jerez-Mayorga, D., & Rios, I. J. C. (2019). Reliability of isometric and isokinetic trunk flexor strength using a functional electromechanical dynamometer. *PeerJ*, 7, e7883. https://doi.org/10.7717/peerj.7883

Santos, E. J., & Silva, J. R. (2022). Force-velocity profiling in sports performance: Practical applications and considerations. *European Journal of Applied Physiology*, 122(2), 353–363.

Schoenfeld, B. J. (2012). Does exercise-induced muscle damage play a role in skeletal muscle hypertrophy? *Journal of Strength and Conditioning Research*, 26(5), 1441–1453. https://doi.org/10.1519/JSC.0b013e31824f207e

Schoenfeld, B. J. (2013). Potential mechanisms for a role of metabolic stress in hypertrophic adaptations to resistance training. *Sports Medicine*, 43(3), 179–194. https://doi.org/10.1007/s40279-013-0017-1

Torres-Banduc, M., Chirosa-Ríos, I. J., Chirosa-Ríos, L., & Jerez-Mayorga, D. (2023). Impact of starting knee flexion angle on muscle activity and performance during plyometrics without jumping. *Sensors*, 24(1), 44.

Wilk, K. E., Arrigo, C. A., & Bagwell, M. S. (2021). Rehabilitation and training with functional electromechanical dynamometry. *Sports Health*, 13(4), 333–343.

Section 2

Assessing Strength in Sport Specific Tasks

5 Dynamometric Technology

Revolutionizing Evaluation and Training in Team Sports

Luis Javier Chirosa Ríos and Ignacio J. Chirosa Rios

Why Talk About Useful Strength in Team Sports?

Brief Conceptual Approach

All training, especially strength training, should be aimed at achieving or maintaining optimal values of useful strength or strength applied in competition gestures.

2000: Chirosa-Ríos et al.

Undoubtedly, the improvement in attack has been preceded by extraordinary evolution in defenses, leading to great specialists who master movements and body control through close marking of their opponents.

2002: González-Badillo and Ribas Serna

We emphasize and insist that strength thus becomes a vitally important physical capacity in handball. It is, in our view, the cornerstone on which the player's physical development relies, significantly influencing their technical-tactical repertoire.

2014: Wagner et al.

The high command of space, the requirement to perform any skill in the shortest possible time, and the employment of maximum speed in decisive actions are variables that will be very present in the game and hence in its preparation. All these factors: space, time, and power, depend on the muscular strength the player can exhibit.

DOI: 10.4324/9781003425182-7

2019: Hermassi et al.

Currently, players are faster, bigger (not necessarily in Spain's case), and stronger, and manage to stay in top form for longer periods.

2019: Büchel et al.

In line with the sport's demands, what interests a handball player is not a disproportionate increase in structural and functional factors, but rather how that strength capacity is transferred and/or applied to the reality of the game. That is, how having adequate muscle development will allow the player to throw faster or jump farther, all while doing so at the right time (temporal adjustment) and in the right situation (spatial adjustment).

20th Century (1990s): Evolution from Behaviorism to Cognitivism

Strength Work: Behaviorist Vision

- **Origin**: Traditional training systems typical of individual sports (athletics, etc.).
- **Key Idea**: Inspired by traditional training systems of individual sports, separation, and independent treatment of factors thought to influence game performance.
- **Consequences**: Technical-tactical preparation was done apart from physical preparation, without considering the type of physical load produced during technical-tactical work.

Strength Work: Cognitivist Vision

- **Origin**: Innovation in understanding strength work applied to handball.
- **Key Idea**: Integration of performance-determining factors into training, making decision-making and the conditional factor extensive to the design and development of any task.
- **Consequences**: Systematic universalization. Fundamental changes in how training and physical preparation are conceived in team sports.

Milestones:

- **Task Classification**: Based on functional relationship with main game gestures (movement, jump, fight, throw) (Seirul-lo, 1987).
- **Integration of Performance Factors in Tasks**: Tasks are designed to incorporate physical, technical, tactical, and psychological components

of performance, ensuring a holistic approach to athlete development (Chirosa-Ríos, 1998).
- **Task Classification**: According to similarity with competition gesture, age, and training stage of the handball player (general, targeted, special, competition) (Martínez et al., 2002).

21st Century

First Decade

Strength Work: Applied Vision

- **Origin**: Exponential development and evolution of methodology and preparation systems in team sports.
- **Key Idea**: Integrated strength training aimed at achieving or maintaining optimal values of strength applied in competition gestures.
- **Consequences**: Use of resistances equal or very close to competition ones. Speed is the determining factor of effort's nature as well as task duration and, consequently, training.

Milestones:

- **Strength Training Programming Foundations**: The principles for effective strength training programming are grounded in scientific and practical approaches to optimize performance and adaptation (González Badillo & Ribas Serna, 2002).

Second Decade

Strength Work: Technological Vision

- **Origin**: Use of new technologies for controlling and monitoring the handball player's preparation process.
- **Key Idea**: Sensory and control of sessions on the field itself, allowing direct monitoring and adjustment of training load.
- **Consequences**: Methodological strategy and regulation based on real-time data from team members (radar, accelerometry, linear encoders, etc.).

Milestones:

- **Physical-Technical-Tactical Tests**: Decision-making and cognitive factor in the scientific assessment of physical condition in team sports (Rivilla-Garcia et al., 2011).

Strength Work: Integrated Dynamometric Vision

- **Origin**: Dynamometric technological innovation.
- **Key Idea**: Stimulus simulation and exhaustive dynamometric control of variables (load, power, speed, inertial factor, space, etc.).
- **Consequences**: Specific development of the desired strength manifestation (static, dynamic, or reactive) in an adjusted, objective, and appropriate manner depending on the season's moment and physical planning.

Milestones:

- **Individualized Determination**: Continuous and dynamic of the acute (intra-session) and accumulated (inter-session) impact of the work done.
- **Optimization Zones/Protection Thresholds**: Knowing, analyzing, and working on each player's force-velocity curves (FVC) allows for designing and practicing personalized methodological strategies without breaking the group's collective dynamics.
- **Task Specificity Optimization**: In relation to the target sports gesture.
- **Continuous Operational State Analysis**: Reducing the risk of injuries and/or illnesses due to overexertion (chronic fatigue and over-training).
- **Big Data**: Objective, systematic, and automated recording of all information related to work done throughout each cycle and/or effective season. This milestone enables the implementation of predictive models to help improve our sport based on evidence from everyday practice.

Dynamic Dynamometric Interaction Paradigm: Deterministic Force-Context Dichotomy

Based on an integrated dynamometric vision (IDV), any knowledgeable reader will have concluded that "strength must not only be proportionally trained." Regardless of the improved performance and effectiveness for real gameplay, it involves observing, analyzing, and determining whether a positive and programmed effect is achieved concerning the CONTEXT in which strength work occurs, thereby achieving maximum transfer and application. Simultaneously, this proportional improvement must be adjusted to each player's structural and functional characteristics, which is crucial for enhancing protection. Any performance improvement will be accompanied by adaptations that imply safety and protection.

IDV allows the use of new technologies with a dual function. On one hand, they are authentic "catalysts" for any programmed process, optimizing and improving its efficiency while acting as "locators," akin to a "GPS" that can always be consulted about our players' true location and whether it matches all variables conditioning the application context (planning, control, and systematization, safety, and communication).

Understanding strength training in handball from a deterministic dichotomous vision of the force-context relationship, utilizing new technologies' assistance, facilitates and speeds up the functions performed by a coach and their professional team. It allows for quickly and safely resolving issues such as planning and organizing work throughout the season, determining where to place elements related to specific strength manifestations and why, evaluating players' improvements, understanding its impact on group or team growth, and considering factors like age and player training. The player takes a central role in this vision and participates in the process, being aware of everything happening.

Ultimately, IDV answers a crucial question that has so far had partial and, in some cases, contradictory answers: "how much and how should we train?" The answer lies in personalized strength training dosing, allowing the administration of "dose-response" strength with the same precision as administering a drug or medication. In this line of thought, the "repetition" is considered the minimum modifiable unit from which to build a task applicable through a specific methodology that respects the established planning.

To facilitate understanding of this reality, the following points in this chapter will address the knowledge, development, and application of what many professionals are beginning to consider the "integrated dynamometric methodology (IDM)" for evaluating, prescribing, and dosing specific strength work in handball. IDV and IDM have allowed and continue to allow exponential growth in scientific and methodological activity in this regard.

This new paradigm, based on the deterministic dichotomy of the reciprocal force-context interaction, posits that all events related to strength work (planning, strategic approach, tasks, etc.) are causally determined by the cause-consequence/dose-response chain. This makes both the future and the past potentially "predictable" from the present as long as we perfectly know our current position in the causality chain. For this reason, many sports science specialists and coaches advocate for the role of new technologies as a useful guide or GPS to inform about this temporal situation.

Integrated Dynamometric Methodology

How to transform any exercise into a useful task for the player?

Any proposal for force-context interaction linked to sports performance must follow a precise methodological sequence starting with the "Design and Definition of the Task."

A task is any exercise that, once analyzed and treated based on the "Practical Systematization Factors" (biomechanics, specificity, muscle, and joint chains), has a specific objective, whether for performance improvement or functional protection of a particular player.

Deepening the understanding and knowledge of the IDM should lead any specialist and professional to a meticulous analysis of the scheme as following this construct reveals the importance of the task and, with it, the repetition as the "Minimum Dynamometric Unit (MDU)" from which to build any stimulus, which will in turn be perfectly situated in the planning and/or training program. For a more detailed understanding of the above, please go through the "Variable Stimulus Methods: New Methodological Proposals for Strength Training" section.

Mastering the methodological bases and factors that allow the "transformation" of any exercise, regardless of its source, into a specific task concerning the moment and subject or subgroup of application allows for continuing to define the dynamometric methodological sequence objectively and balanced.

Integrated Dynamometric Methodology: Designing the "Method-Task" Binomial

IDM for the correct design of the "Method-Task" binomial involves combining specific training methodologies with highly targeted tasks focusing on dynamometric performance, that is, real-time measurement of the strength of the muscles or muscle groups involved. This approach aims to optimize training through personalization based on precise and objective data, improving both the effectiveness and efficiency of the training process.

Defining the Force Expressions and Type of Contraction

It is crucial to be intentional and strict when defining the type of strength manifestations and the type of contraction we want to train and improve during each session.

Related to strength manifestations, regardless of existing classifications in selected literature (Vittori, 1990; González-Badillo & Ribas Serna, 2002), what really interests the trainer is where to focus the stimulus, that is, on which part of the FVC, performance improvement is sought to ensure the greatest and best transfer to actions that are crucial within the real game (execution speed, throw precision, jump reach, and amplitude). These aspects will be addressed in more detail in the "Determining the Training Zone" section.

Undoubtedly, solving this section involves answering with certainty the questions: why is it being trained? and what is the purpose or focus of such training? The way the training is oriented is called the "Training Perspective". It is essential to analyze, select, and know what the final objectives are at each moment of the planning to be developed (Structural—Functional—Cognitive—Therapeutic) since, depending on how the training is oriented, the short and medium-term goals and objectives will be conditioned, allowing for a specific adaptation that must be perfectly aligned with the individual planning of each player and, therefore, with the collective and general planning of the team.

Next, a brief description of each perspective in which strength methods are aligned will be provided:

Structural Perspective

This perspective's main objective is to increase the muscle's cross-sectional area. The adaptations sought are primarily morphological. Within this perspective, there is a subdivision determined by the intention to move the assigned external resistance at maximum possible speed or controlled speed. Here lies the key and the emphasis should be made. The crucial factor is determining if the movement is performed at maximum speed. From this point, variables like time under tension and the magnitude of the displaced resistance come into play. The first variable is linked to metabolic stress, and the second to mechanical stress. The objectives of these approaches can be aesthetic or, in specific health cases, functional.

For handball players, increasing the cross-sectional area for health and protection purposes may be of interest but never for aesthetic purposes. Occasionally, this type of training can be done at certain moments of the player's training, as well as in specific recovery sessions for already fully trained players. When working on this structural perspective, the focus should generally be on improving strength by stimulating selective hypertrophy. This is achieved by intending to move the load at maximum speed, but it is also essential to consider if the effort is performed until total fatigue or not (in the latter case, it will be said that the effort character is being worked on) (González-Badillo & Ribas Serna, 2002; Sánchez-Medina & González-Badillo, 2011). In a handball player, the tendency should be toward improving explosive (active and reactive) strength and optimizing segmental speed. Therefore, the importance of not provoking or doing hypertrophy just to develop bigger players is emphasized. There is a risk of making the player larger but also potentially harmful by requiring them to move a muscle mass that is not functional, achieving the opposite effect.

One must consider the player profile to be developed, as the specific position played regularly will be a crucial aspect to consider. The muscle gains achieved will be in line with the specific position's requirements. For example, a "first-line" player will have a different work orientation than a pivot. In both cases, structural strength training must focus on selective hypertrophy, mainly targeting fast fibers IIx and IIa, resulting in strength production improvements without losing efficiency in the overall motor dynamics associated with the game.

Functional Perspective

This perspective seeks to improve neural factors; in summary, the strength gains (in their different expressions—both N·s and N·m) are due in all cases to optimizing any neural factors involved in strength production (recruitment, synchronization, co-activation, etc.). Nowadays, the term "functional" is confused with using exercises with more coordinative or balance connotation. Still, when referring to this training perspective, we mean improving strength production through neural adaptations.

The terms should not be confused. In reality, the goal is to improve force production per unit of time, and for this, it is necessary that the athlete's structures can develop those high levels of strength and withstand the mechanical stress generated in this training perspective. This includes methods with high loads to work with bodyweight, such as multi-jumps or intensive plyometrics. As mentioned, the determining factor of these methods is the relationship between the strength and the time it is applied, which is very short. Therefore, it must be clear that whenever functional perspective training is mentioned, these two key factors will be referenced. However, in the case of strength training in this perspective for our sport, the aspect of "variability" and "continuous adjustment" to the multiple conditions that will occur throughout any technical-tactical element (continuous space-time adjustment) must also be considered. Ultimately, the goal is to throw faster in changing time intervals, run faster adjusted to often undefined space (due to the opponent's variable and random performance), make explosive directional changes with variability and uncertainty, jump higher, etc., all while adhering to the logic of the game where precise tactical adjustment determines the final performance.

Cognitive Perspective

Focused on selecting, integrating, and developing decision-making strategies during specific strength training, this perspective is considered a fundamental pillar in the handball player's training. The logic of this form of work relies on common sense and intuition, as there is insufficient scientific literature to demonstrate its effectiveness. There is a lack of experimental studies demonstrating reciprocal strength gains and simultaneous decision-making improvement.

The execution procedure is simple. To facilitate understanding, as a practical example, a typical task like a Dumbbell Bench Press is selected. A teammate positions themselves visibly for the player executing the Press, indicating which arm to perform the Press with through either a specific stimulus or a general cue like a number.

Working with strategies analogous to the cognitive perspective, it can be inferred that the neuromotor system is activated in a manner more similar to the cognitive demands of real gameplay. This approach opens windows in the motor cortex, increasing brain plasticity and fostering the development of players who can respond to open, more creative, and game-need-adjusted behaviors.

Therapeutic Perspective

Advancements in training theory knowledge have been accompanied by improvements in players' physical condition. Concurrently, this has led to a gradual increase in competitive requirements and demands, along with a growing number of high-intensity matches, resulting in a higher injury risk. This increasingly demanding reality sometimes leads to player injuries, causing multifactorial negative impacts from the perspective of physical preparation, loss of training hours, motivational perspective, player frustration, and finally, from an institutional perspective, the consequent economic cost and the risk of not meeting the scheduled sports objectives.

Given this, it is necessary to create training strategies that promote protection. These strategies are dynamic and closely related to each season's moment, allowing players to be individually placed on a "balance" between conditional improvement or optimization and functional or therapeutic protection. Evaluating, analyzing, and working synergistically and integrally on aspects related to physical condition and sensoriomotor-proprioceptive systems allow reaching thresholds aligned with what can be termed each player's "Individual Protection Zone."

In summary, the therapeutic perspective involves planning works that promote player protection, through either compensatory strength tasks for synergistic and antagonistic muscles or tasks that stimulate lateral balance. Handball is a sport where gestures like throwing or jumping involve unbalanced lateralities, meaning there may be muscular imbalances that cause or favor injury events-mechanisms. This invites the development of so-called mirror tasks, a set of specific compensatory exercises where proprioception or improvement of the sensoriomotor system plays a fundamental role. The goal is to protect the athlete and prevent potential injuries due to systematic practice of our sport.

Determining the Training Zone

We are now at the "Methodological Funnel with FEMD" (progression toward maximum specificity) moment, where maximum emphasis must be placed on adjusting the individualized stimulus. To achieve this, it is essential to have means to train with exhaustive control of the speed, force, or power developed in each repetition. When the goal is to maximize the stimulus's effect applied in static or static-dynamic manifestations, it is necessary to know the optimal relationship between force and time. In dynamic manifestations, it is essential to know the load (force) and the speed at which it is moved, or the optimal power developed.

To facilitate and simplify the analysis and understanding of "Training Zones," a scale has been designed on the "FVC." This tool allows for orderly management of load organization and control.

When referring to "Training Zones," we mean those bands or intervals within the "FVC" in relation to the spectrum of external loads or resistances to be moved by pushing or holding the external resistance. The "1RM" or 100% of "Maximum Dynamic Force (MDF)" as a reference for maximum intensity for the general training context. This manifestation should be called concentric MDF or "MDFc" since when evaluated with free weights, the predominant muscular action is usually pushing. Therefore, it is essential to recognize two fundamental strategies for force production. The first is exhibited when pushing an external resistance or applying force against gravity, known as pushing (P). The second occurs when holding or resisting an external load, known as holding (H), which includes stopping the force of gravity (Schaefer et al., 2023).

Thus, if we control and know the stimulus's nature, it is easy to identify which adaptation will be achieved. Applying a method that allows working under optimal conditions to achieve the set goals becomes a logical, systematic, and automated process. It is the quickest and safest way for our players to train and, more importantly, compete under programmed and controlled mechanical-metabolic-coordinative demands, fulfilling the adaptation principle and the optimization-protection rule.

In any case, the way to progress in developing specific strength is under the structural adaptation construct. This means that to move up a level in function, the structures must be prepared to withstand the higher tension and demands of the new functional level desired.

The possibilities are considerable; the key is determining which zone of the FVC the training focuses on. This will produce a specific adaptation that favors evolution toward a higher functional level facilitating adaptations toward improving specific strength. Initially, ten clearly differentiated zones are identified regarding strength training method organization and classification.

Execution and Control

Execution, that is, the enactment of everything previously outlined and controlling those actions, is the final step. Now it is about verifying the appropriateness of the proposed tasks and the effect they are having on our athletes.

It is crucial that different team members have a high sense of responsibility when planning and systematically recording each season's progress and incidents, verifying the effect of each method used on individual and collective player performance. All of this is essential to do using the scientific method to ensure the results' validity. This is the way to favor decision-making between periods, promoting continuous growth for both players and the technical team.

Using IDM and new technologies makes it easy to understand that load quantification and control are key. Through training monitoring, the knowledge of what the immediate and accumulated training responses are gained concretely and precisely. This ensures the athlete's effective evolution, knowing their current form state (operational state), and clearly reduces the risk of overuse injuries (chronic fatigue and over-training states) (Gabbett, 2016). Drew and Finch (2016) indicate in a systematic review that there is currently specific scientific evidence associating training load and injury or illness risk, recommending, if not demanding, exhaustive workload control to reduce future unnecessary risks.

How to Create Methods to Improve Strength in Team Sports

There are numerous strength training method proposals in the general sports field, and classifications are innumerable, creating confusion among professionals. From our perspective, a method is the perfect combination of the task (t) and the programmed stimulus (m), considering the pursued objective with the selected perspective and the training zone to be used.

A method (m) would be well-defined if the task (t) has been correctly selected-designed, and on the other hand, all the differentiating elements of the stimulus, perspective, and training zone have been justly chosen. This is what we have called in our vision the application of the "INTEGRATED DYNAMOMETRIC METHODOLOGY."

The real challenge lies in translating these concepts from the theoretical to the theoretical-practical or directly practical plane without requiring excessive effort from coaches or athletes. Therefore, the next section will detail the essential keys to effectively implementing this training methodology in daily practice. This process will facilitate a deeper understanding and more effective application of training techniques, ensuring professionals and athletes can maximize their results efficiently and sustainably.

Practical Case: Application of Integrated Dynamometric Methodology

To understand the IDM steps, we will use the example of a "first-line" player whose structural base we want to improve without losing explosiveness. First (1), we need to analyze which group or set of actions we want to impact: (a) fight actions, (b) movement, (c) jump, or (d) throw. Suppose we want to improve their jump capacity in both vertical and horizontal vectors. For this, we will select tasks (t) that impact the lower body's musculature. Next (2), we will choose the method (m) in which, on the one hand, we will have to select the perspective (3). As mentioned, morphological or structural factors are desired to improve, so the structural perspective will be chosen, and since gestural explosiveness or speed should not be lost, we will work in the "Neural-Morphological (MN)" training zone (4).

The stimuli for a programmed session of a specific exercise could be: 5 series of an "x" number of repetitions, maintaining a speed threshold above 90% of average speed, with 2-minute active recoveries between series. The working forms regarding the type of external resistance used could be multiple if using a FEMD. If using other technology like an accelerometer, resistance could be variable (elastic bands in multiple planes); in the case of a linear encoder, it limits the use to more stable resistances like free weights in one plane or inertial if using a rotational encoder, allowing work in multiple planes at the expense of control of manifested force. The problem in these two cases is the indirect or estimated force calculation, as with this type of technology, an external fixed load must always be selected, and there is no force sensor (the main advantage of FEMD, as the system itself generates the load and calculates the manifested force).

Without going into excessive detail, strength training planning for handball, soccer, basketball, and so forth should progress from more global and non-specific work in the early training stages, primarily developing structural and protection aspects, to functional-cognitive work along with their mirror protection tasks in the specialization stage. This scheme applies not only to the training process but also to planning at all levels.

As a general rule, during the preparatory period, structural perspective volume is higher than during competitive periods, just as when starting a microcycle, allowing for greater orientation in this sense than at the end of it, where functional, cognitive, and protection perspectives must be more than present. Therefore, it is a continuum that coaches and trainers must be aware of, considering the players' individual differences, where besides personal characteristics, other factors like specific position, learning level, or acquired mastery, or accumulated practice years will influence.

The player's maturation related to strength training will condition the athlete to acquire a morpho-functional structure that allows them to respond successfully to game demands. The limitation in any case may be caused by a phenomenon known as the "ceiling effect," meaning the person has reached their expression limits of any technical-tactical skill or physical quality. A strategy followed to solve this problem and avoid stagnation or decline is using new methodological proposals, emphasizing stimulus variation and similarity with the sports gesture (principles of variability and specificity).

In the last decade, multiple interesting methodological proposals have emerged, applying these two training principles. These trends have been accompanied by scientific research demonstrating their effectiveness (Baena Morales, 2016). The next section will present the main proposals within the known methods as Intra-repetition Variable Stimulus Methods (MEVIR).

Intra-repetition Variable Stimulus Methods: New Methodological Proposals for Strength Training

The search for specificity and improvement of practical strategies in strength training favoring adaptation, especially in experienced players, has led to new paradigms based on stimulus variation during different phases of a repetition, known as variable stimulus methods in both series and intra-repetition (MEVIR) (Chirosa-Ríos et al., 2014). According to a recent review, variable stimulus training can produce greater adaptations in various strength manifestations (Suchomel et al., 2018).

Among the different ways of proposing variable stimulus work are those established by Chirosa-Ríos et al. (2014), summarized next.

Variable Resistance "Between Series"

Resistance is modified between series of a training session. For example, a traditional strength session with different strength exercises like bench press, squats, and so forth, followed by a session with multi-jumps or the same session with more or less load or volume. Chirosa-Ríos (1998) conducted a study showing that this type of combination improved jump capacity in study subjects.

Variable Resistance "Intra Series"

Resistance is modified within the same series being performed. For example, a series with 4 repetitions of squats at 80% (1RM) followed by 6 repetitions at 30% (1RM). This type of work, when adequate time is allowed between the overloaded series and the light series, produces a phenomenon called post-activation potentiation. This training method is also known as contrast or complex training, working the same way by combining heavy load strength work with lighter or explosive methods. If enough time is allowed to avoid fatigue and not dissipate the effects, it will improve the neuromuscular capacity to produce strength and greater dynamic transfer to the competition gesture with higher training density.

Variable Resistance "Between Repetitions"

Resistance is modified between repetitions of the same series. An example of variable resistance "between repetitions" (VRBR) is performing one repetition with 90% of the RM and the other three of the series with 45%. It must be considered that variable resistance intra-repetition (VRIR) and variable resistance intra-set (VRIS) would mean a resistance variation at the same time, as varying resistance within the series is similar to doing it between repetitions; the difference lies in the waiting time, which produces the potentiation. Here, the mechanism is different and more related to synchronization processes.

Variable Resistance "Intra-Repetition"

Resistance changes within the same repetition being performed. In this case, the aim is to modify the stimulus within the same repetition. This training type is increasingly used and has strong scientific support (Granados et al., 2007; Saeterbakken et al., 2011). The benefits include greater neuro-muscular activation and consequently an increase in muscular demand, producing strength and power improvement more than traditional training using only free weights (Chirosa-Ríos et al., 2014).

Examples for working VRIR include stato-dynamic methods, producing isometric phases within a concentric or eccentric phase. Works have also been carried out where load implementation within the repetition using chains or elastic bands within traditional exercises can alter an exercise's load profile by modifying the way force is produced during movement. For example, placing an elastic band can modify the end of the eccentric phase and the end of the concentric phase, which may or may not coincide with mechanical efficiency points.

The emergence of new technologies applied to the strength field has facilitated the use of variable resistance (VR) in general and VRIR in particular as new training models applied to sports performance, especially in athletes close to their maximum strength and needing new individualized and personalized stimuli impacting various internal factors modulating force production.

To conclude and attempt to summarize the concept of functional electromechanical dynamometry (FEMD), as its name suggests, it is associated with using an electronic dynamometer controlled by software to generate external stimuli of any kind. This means that this technology can simulate any device or equipment on the market for strength work (free weights, inertial devices like conical pulley or yoyo, elastic bands or chains, isokinetic devices, vibrating machines) with the advantage of having all this in the same space. Another virtue is having immediate data and feedback, facilitating learning in specific tasks where information will help the player modulate force application as needed.

Practically speaking, the most interesting aspect is that training can be performed according to the effort character, ending the series once the repetition does not reach the established force or speed ranges for the task. Practical versatility is maximal, allowing training from multiple perspectives. Knowing what is to be achieved and having the imagination to design situations fitting the season moment and each player's characteristics is necessary. Applied stimuli can practically reproduce any action or effort desired to be represented. The challenge now is knowing the effect of stimuli that could not be controlled and understanding their impact on our athletes, even generating stimuli previously unknown to trainers and sports science specialists. It can be concluded that we are at the start of a new era in sports and health sciences.

References

Baena Morales, S. (2016). *Análisis Comparativo Del Press de Banca Utilizando Métodos de Fuerza Con y Sin Resistencia Variable Intra-Repetición.* Granada: Universidad de Granada, http://hdl.handle.net/10481/43838

Büchel, D., Jakobsmeyer, R., Döring, M., Adams, M., Rückert, U., & Baumeister, J. (2019). Effect of Playing Position and Time On-Court on Activity Profiles in German Elite Team Handball. *International Journal of Performance Analysis in Sport*, *19*(5), 832–844. https://doi.org/10.1080/24748668.2019.1663071

Chirosa-Ríos, I. J., Baena, S., Soria-gila, M. Á., Bautista, I. J., & Chirosa, L. J. (2014). Intra-Repetition Variable Resistance Training: Part 1 An Overview. *European Journal of Human Movement*, *32*, 48–60.

Chirosa-Ríos, L. J. (1998). *Entrenamiento con un método de contraste para la mejora de la fuerza de impulsion en relación a otro de tipo convencional en balonmano*. Tesis Doctora. Universidad de Granada.

Chirosa-Ríos, L. J., Ríos, I. C., & Padial, P. (2000). Efecto Del Entrenamiento Integrado Sobre La Mejora de La Fuerza de Impulsión En Un Lanzamiento En Suspensión En Balonmano. *European Journal of Human Movement*, (6), 155–174. https://dialnet.unirioja.es/servlet/articulo?codigo=2278414&info=resumen&idioma=ENG

Drew, M. K., & Finch, C. F. (2016). The Relationship Between Training Load and Injury, Illness and Soreness: A Systematic and Literature Review. *Sports Medicine*, *46*(6), 861–883. https://doi.org/10.1007/s40279-015-0459-8

Gabbett, T. J. (2016). The Training—Injury Prevention Paradox: Should Athletes Be Training Smarter and Harder? *British Journal of Sports Medicine*, *50*(5), 273–280. https://doi.org/10.1136/BJSPORTS-2015-095788

González-Badillo, J. J., & Ribas Serna, J. (2002). *Bases de la Programación del entrenamiento de fuerza*. Barcelona, España: Inde.

Granados, C., Izquierdo, M., Ibañez, J., Bonnabau, H., & Gorostiaga, E. M. (2007). Differences in Physical Fitness and Throwing Velocity Among Elite and Amateur Female Handball Players. *International Journal of Sports Medicine*, *28*(10), 860–867. https://doi.org/10.1055/s-2007-964989

Hermassi, S., Wollny, R., Schwesig, R., Shephard, R. J., & Chelly, M. S. (2019). Effects of In-Season Circuit Training on Physical Abilities in Male Handball Players. *Journal of Strength and Conditioning Research*, *33*(4), 944–957. https://doi.org/10.1519/JSC.0000000000002270

Martínez, I., Cuadrado-Sáenz, G., & Paz, J. (2002). *El Entrenamiento De La Fuerza Mediante Autocargas*. II Congreso Internacional de La Asociación Española de Ciencias Del Deporte, Madrid, Del 14 Al 16 de Marzo Del 2002, 1–12.

Rivilla-Garcia, J., Grande Rodriguez, I., Sampedro, J., & van den Tillaar, R. (2011). Influence of Opposition on Ball Velocity in the Handball Jump Throw. *Journal of Sports Science and Medicine*, *10*(3), 534–539.

Saeterbakken, A. H., van den Tillaar, R., & Seiler, S. (2011). Effect of Core Stability Training on Throwing. *Journal of Strength and Conditioning Research*, *25*(3), 712–718.

Sánchez-Medina, L., & González-Badillo, J. J. (2011). Velocity Loss as an Indicator of Neuromuscular Fatigue During Resistance Training. *Medicine and Science in Sports and Exercise*, *43*(9), 1725–1734. https://doi.org/10.1249/MSS.0b013e318213f880

Schaefer, L. V., Carnarius, F., Dech, S., & Bittmann, F. N. (2023). Repeated Measurements of Adaptive Force: Maximal Holding Capacity Differs from Other Maximal Strength Parameters and Preliminary Characteristics for Non-Professional Strength vs. Endurance Athletes. *Frontiers in Physiology*, *14*, 1020954.

Seirul-lo, F. (1987). Opción de planificación en los deportes de largo período de competiciones. *Revista de Entrenamiento Deportivo*, *3*(3), 53–62. www.entrenamientodeportivo.org/articulos/plan_dep_largo_per_comp_fsv.pdf

Suchomel, T. J., Nimphius, S., Bellon, C. R., & Stone, M. H. (2018). The Importance of Muscular Strength: Training Considerations. *Sports Medicine*, *48*(4), 765–785. https://doi.org/10.1007/s40279-018-0862-z

Vittori, C. (1990). El entrenamiento de la fuerza para el sprint. *RED*, *4*(3), 2–8.

Wagner, H., Pfusterschmied, P., Tilp, M., Landlinger, J., von Duvillard, S. P., & Müller, E. (2014). Upper-Body Kinematics in Team-Handball Throw, Tennis Serve, and Volleyball Spike. *Scandinavian Journal of Medicine & Science in Sports*, *24*(2), 345–354. https://doi.org/10.1111/j.1600-0838.2012.01503.x

6 Assessment of Strength in Sports Tasks

Darío Martínez-García and Luis Javier Chirosa Ríos

Introduction

Sports sciences are continually advancing with the progress of technology, and at the forefront of these developments is the assessment of athletes' physical capabilities (Issurin 2010). A critical aspect of this assessment is the evaluation of strength in specific sporting gestures. Strength, an essential component of athletic performance, is not merely a measure of muscle power but rather a complex interplay of force, velocity, and endurance, tailored to meet the demands of various sports activities (Kraemer and Ratamess 2004).

The introduction of functional electromechanical dynamometers (FEMD) represents a significant advancement in this field. These devices provide precise, reliable, and sport-specific assessments of muscular strength, rendering them indispensable tools for sports science professionals (Rodriguez-Perea et al. 2021). Their applications extend from optimizing training protocols to supporting injury prevention and rehabilitation efforts.

The importance of strength assessment in sports cannot be overstated. It plays a crucial role in identifying areas for potential improvement, ensuring that athletes achieve their peak performance levels while also mitigating the risk of sport-related injuries (Bourne et al. 2018). FEMDs are pivotal in this process, delivering accurate measurements of muscle strength and endurance across various joints and movements. This encompasses key athletic gestures such as jumping, throwing, and changes of direction, each requiring distinct muscular engagements and force manifestations.

Furthermore, the dynamometer's role in elucidating the manifestations of force in sports gestures—such as maximal force, power, rate of force development (RFD), and impulse—is indispensable. These force manifestations are critical indicators of an athlete's capacity to perform specific sports actions both effectively and safely.

In this chapter, we will explore the specifics of major athletic gestures, examine various methodologies for their evaluation, and conclude by discussing the significance of these assessments in the broader context of sports performance and injury prevention.

DOI: 10.4324/9781003425182-8

Main Athletic Gestures and Their Measurements

Relevance of Assessments in Sport Performance

The precise assessment of strength in athletic performance is a key point of effective sport intervention and injury prevention programs (Cerda Vega et al. 2018). The advancement of FEMD represents a significant leap forward in our ability to not only obtain valid and reliable muscular strength data but also achieve practical and specific measurements across a variety of athletic gestures. These assessments are essential for a comprehensive understanding of an athlete's current physical capabilities, thereby guiding the development of tailored training regimens, rehabilitation protocols, and performance enhancement strategies (García-Buendía et al. 2022).

Recent technological advancements, such as FEMDs and artificial intelligence, have catalyzed a paradigm shift in the methodology of strength measurement. These innovations include improvements in sensor accuracy, data processing algorithms, and user interfaces, making these devices more intuitive and effective for sports scientists and coaches. Detailed analyses play a pivotal role in crafting bespoke training and rehabilitation programs, addressing the nuanced needs of athletes across a diverse array of sports disciplines.

The predominant methodology in sports performance evaluation has traditionally involved a combination of isolated objective data points, such as one-repetition maximum (1RM) and the velocity-based training (VBT) of general, analytical, or sport-specific exercises, alongside subjective variables like the rating of perceived exertion (RPE) (Garcia-Ramos et al. 2018). These individual metrics, however, offer only a fragmented view of an athlete's overall condition. Coaches are often compelled to develop their own databases in an attempt to integrate all available measurements, striving to create a more comprehensive evaluation and prediction of an athlete's performance.

While such methodologies provide valuable insights, they fall short in delivering a holistic picture of an athlete's readiness and potential (Turner et al. 2019). The disjointed nature of these data points often leads to gaps in understanding, making it difficult to accurately assess an athlete's true performance capabilities or injury risk.

In response to these limitations, the integration of advanced tools like FEMD enable a more cohesive approach to performance evaluation, allowing for the synthesis of both objective and subjective data into a unified framework. By leveraging these technologies, coaches and sports scientists can gain deeper insights into an athlete's performance, leading to more precise training adaptations and injury prevention strategies.

Until recently, the integration of discrete data points—such as maximal strength, peak power, and range of motion—offered a somewhat broader understanding of the technical gestures relevant to a specific sport. However, this approach still provided only a partial view of an athlete's performance capabilities. In response, a "complex systems approach" has been introduced to describe intricate problems in fields such as medicine, biology, economics, and social sciences (Bittencourt et al. 2016). This novel approach could offer fresh insights into complex issues like sports performance and injury incidence. The interactive units within a complex system form a network of determining factors where variables interact often chaotically and unpredictably by nowadays methods. Essentially, it is not a single variable that should be evaluated but rather the intricate interplay between intrinsic and extrinsic factors, both modifiable and non-modifiable.

In this context, sports performance or injury prediction within the "athlete system" emerges as a complex model, necessitating the measurement of most variables inherent to a sports gesture. The sequence of data obtained within a single repetition—such as rate of RFD, strength, power, work, and impulse (both mean and maximum) across concentric, eccentric, and isometric phases—provides revealing information (Rodriguez-Perea et al. 2021). These metrics, although often underexplored, could indeed offer a more accurate reflection of an athlete's reality and performance.

Rather than focusing on isolated variables, this method acknowledges the multifaceted nature of athletic performance, where numerous factors interact in dynamic and non-linear ways. By embracing this perspective, coaches and sports scientists can develop more sophisticated models that better capture the true complexity of athletic performance. This not only enhances the accuracy of performance assessments but also improves the ability to tailor interventions that are more closely aligned with the unique needs of each athlete, ultimately leading to better performance outcomes and reduced injury risk.

In this sense, Greig and Langley (2024) contributed to the discourse by examining the functionality of dynamometry, in the biomechanical analysis of movement. Their study's objective to align isokinetic testing protocols with the functional goals of rehabilitation or sports performance led to innovative findings. By analyzing walking gait and establishing specific concentric and eccentric demands for knee movements, the research underscored the potential of these devices to inform more tailored, functionally relevant data collection protocols. This approach not only elevates the clinical and training relevance of FEMD assessments but also emphasizes the dynamometer's adaptability to specific rehabilitative needs and performance enhancement goals.

Athletic Gestures

Across the wide array of sports disciplines, there are certain athletic gestures that, while adapted to the specific demands of each sport, recur with some consistency across various activities:

Jumping

An athletic gesture that, regardless of the sport, aims to propel the athlete's body into a flight phase. Both the take-off and landing phases of a jump engage key muscle groups, including the quadriceps, hamstrings, glutes, adductors, and calves. The ability to generate optimal power through the coordinated action of these muscles is crucial in sports such as long jump, high jump, basketball, and volleyball, among others (Ramirez-Campillo et al. 2020).

The effectiveness of a jump, be it for height or distance, relies heavily on the precise timing and synergy of muscle contractions. For instance, in basketball, the explosive power generated by these muscle groups can make the difference between a successful dunk and a missed opportunity, while in volleyball, it is essential for achieving effective spikes and blocks.

Running

This movement involves a more complex interaction of the lower body muscles. The coordination of the quadriceps, hamstrings, and calves, along with the stabilization of the trunk, is crucial. The effectiveness and synergy of these muscles significantly influence an athlete's speed, endurance, and agility (Garcia-Pinillos et al. 2017).

The quadriceps and hamstrings are primarily responsible for the propulsion and control of leg movement, while the calves contribute to the force applied during the push-off phase. Simultaneously, the core muscles, including the abdominals and lower back, provide the necessary stabilization to maintain balance and posture throughout the running motion.

Efficient running technique hinges on the harmonious function of these muscle groups. For instance, in sprinting, the explosive power of the quadriceps and hamstrings is vital for quick acceleration, whereas in distance running, the emphasis shifts towards endurance, requiring sustained muscle activity over prolonged periods. Agility, another critical component, depends on the athlete's ability to quickly and smoothly change direction, which in turn demands precise muscle coordination and strength.

The efficiency of these muscles directly impacts energy expenditure (Ruiz-Alias et al. 2024). Runners with better muscle coordination and synergy are able to maintain higher speeds with less effort, reducing fatigue and improving overall performance. These types of performance characteristics can be best observed in the generated graphs derived from simulated running evaluations where the focus is on ground contact time and the concentric-excentric interface.

Overhead Throwing

Common in sports such as baseball and javelin, the focus shifts to the upper body. In these actions, the muscles of the shoulder, elbow, and wrist—particularly the rotator cuff muscles, deltoids, and triceps—play a crucial role in generating power and ensuring precision in the throw (Wagner et al. 2012).

The rotator cuff muscles are vital for stabilizing the shoulder joint, allowing for controlled and powerful arm movements, while the deltoids contribute to the lifting and rotational motions of the arm in the cocking phase. The triceps, responsible for extending the elbow, provide the final thrust needed to propel the object with speed and accuracy.

Moreover, the repetitive nature of overhead throwing places significant stress on the shoulder joint and surrounding musculature, making it susceptible to overuse injuries (Cools et al. 2020). As such, targeted strength and conditioning programs are essential not only for enhancing performance but also for preventing injuries. Evaluations that measure and improve the strength, range of motion, and stiffness of the rotator cuff, deltoids, and triceps can help athletes maintain peak performance while minimizing the risk of injury.

Traction

In traction-based sports, such as rock climbing, emphasis is placed on grip strength, the force generated by the back musculature, and eccentric endurance. These sports underscore the critical importance of opposing the force exerted by one's own body weight or the force generated by an opponent (López-Rivera and González-Badillo 2012).

The muscles of the forearm, particularly the flexors, are heavily engaged in sustaining grip in different sport such as judo, rock climbing, of even in shooting sports. This continuous exertion requires not only raw strength but also exceptional endurance to maintain performance over extended periods.

The back muscles, including the latissimus dorsi, trapezius, and rhomboids, are also crucial. Additionally, eccentric strength—the ability to control muscle elongation under tension—is vital to manage a controlled gesture, the muscles must effectively resist the force of gravity to prevent injury.

Stabilization

Stabilization is a fundamental aspect of all sports. Core stability, achieved through the engagement of the abdominal muscles, lower back (lumbar) muscles, and obliques, provides the essential support required for many athletic movements (Reyes-Ferrada et al. 2022).

Core stability is the foundation upon which athletic performance is built. The muscles of the core act as a stabilizing force, enabling athletes to maintain balance, posture, and control during complex movements. Whether it's maintaining a strong stance in combat sports, executing a powerful swing in golf, or controlling body movements during gymnastics, a stable core is indispensable.

Incorporating core stability exercises into training regimes is vital for athletes across all disciplines. Strengthening these muscle groups not only enhances performance but also plays a key role in injury prevention. Weakness or instability in the core can lead to compensatory movements that increase the risk of injury, particularly in the lower back and hips (Reyes-Ferrada et al. 2021).

To sum up, the role of advanced training tools and methodologies, such as FEMDs, becomes particularly valuable. These tools allow for the precise assessment and enhancement of the specific muscle groups or movements involved in these gestures, leading to more effective training programs that can be tailored to the unique demands of each sport.

The real challenge for strength and conditioning coaches is to have a clear mental scheme where they can take advantage of the facilities that are presented to them for the analysis of the specific kinetic chains of each gesture. The implementation and continuous updating of the advantages of this type of evaluation will be reflected in the following benefits.

Functional Applicability: The capacity to replicate movements encountered in daily life and sport, enhanced by customized protocols for data collection. This capability ensures that assessments of muscular performance are not only precise but also directly relevant to the practical demands of athletic and everyday activities.

Enhancement of Rehabilitation and Injury Prevention: By delivering exact and consistent measurements of strength and movement velocity, the FEMD enables the design of personalized training programs. These programs are instrumental in fostering efficient recovery processes while also substantially reducing the likelihood of injuries. The precision of FEMD measurements ensures that rehabilitation efforts can be optimally directed to meet the specific recovery needs of individuals.

Optimization of Athletic Performance: The FEMD's data serves as a critical resource for athletes and their coaching teams, allowing for the meticulous calibration of training strategies. By concentrating on distinct profiles of strength and velocity that are most beneficial for an athlete's performance, the FEMD facilitates a strategic approach to training that is designed to enhance overall athletic output.

Specific Assessment of Athletic Gestures in FEMD

The FEMD offers unparalleled precision in the assessment of athletic gestures, allowing for the recording of force data every millisecond throughout the entire movement. By leveraging its various modes—Isotonic, Isokinetic, Inertial, Isometric, Elastic, and Vibration—coaches and sports scientists can create sport-specific assessments that provide actionable insights into an athlete's performance and areas for improvement.

Jumping

Jumping is a fundamental athletic gesture in many sports. FEMD provides a deep analysis for sports scientists and coaches aiming to enhance vertical jump performance and reduce injury risks.

Proposed Evaluation:

- **Mode:** *Isotonic and Inertial*
- **Objective:** Evaluate and optimize power, force production, and momentum during vertical jumps.
- **Protocol:**
    - **Isotonic Mode:** Utilize the FEMD in isotonic mode to simulate loaded and unloaded jump squats. This mode allows for the assessment of the force generated during both the concentric (take-off) and eccentric (landing) phases of the jump.
    - **Inertial Mode:** Apply the inertial mode to assess the athlete's ability to generate force against varying resistance levels. This is particularly useful for evaluating the momentum developed during the jump, which has been shown to be a critical factor in determining optimal training loads.
- **Analysis:**
    - **Force and Power Output:** Measure the peak power and force generated during the take-off phase. High peak power output is crucial for achieving greater jump heights, a key performance indicator in sports requiring explosive leg strength.
    - **Momentum-Based Load Prescription:** Recent research by Harry et al. (2022) highlights the importance of using system momentum—calculated as the product of the athlete's mass and take-off velocity—as a key metric for prescribing training loads. This approach is superior to traditional velocity-based metrics because it better accounts for the combined effect of load and movement velocity, providing a more accurate assessment of the stimulus on the neuromuscular system.
    - **Eccentric Control and Landing Mechanics:** Assess the force generated during the eccentric phase to evaluate the athlete's control during landing. Poor landing mechanics can lead to increased injury risk, particularly in the knee joint, which is subjected to significant biomechanical stress during jumping activities.
- **Application:**
    - **Training Load Optimization:** The insights from momentum-based load prescriptions can be used to fine-tune the resistance applied during jump squat training, ensuring that the athlete trains at an intensity that maximizes power output without compromising movement velocity.
    - **Injury Prevention and Rehabilitation:** The FEMD's ability to precisely measure eccentric control and landing forces allows for the early identification of biomechanical inefficiencies that could predispose athletes to injuries, such as anterior cruciate ligament (ACL) tears (Bencke

et al. 2013). By addressing these issues through targeted strength and conditioning programs, the risk of injury can be significantly reduced.

- **Performance Enhancement:** Regular monitoring of jumping mechanics with the FEMD can guide the progression of training loads and techniques, helping athletes to continually improve their vertical jump height and overall explosive power. The integration of momentum-based metrics ensures that training is both effective and specific to the athlete's needs.

Running

Running, particularly in sports like football and athletics, places significant biomechanical stress on the knee joint. The coordination of the quadriceps, hamstrings, and calves, along with the stabilization of the trunk, is critical for achieving optimal speed, endurance, and agility. The FEMD enables detailed assessments of these dynamics, providing insights essential for both performance enhancement and injury prevention.

Proposed Evaluation:

- **Mode:** *Inertial and Isokinetic*
- **Objective:** Evaluate quadriceps-hamstring dynamics, force production, and muscle coordination during sprinting and running motions.
- **Protocol:**
    - **Inertial Mode:** Simulate sprinting resistance to assess the athlete's ability to produce force rapidly and maintain speed. This mode is also used to assess how added loads (ranging from 0% to 30% of body weight) affect specific technique and ground contact time.
    - **Isokinetic Mode:** Examine knee extension and flexion under controlled speeds to evaluate the balance between quadriceps and hamstring strength. This mode is also used to assess how different velocities affect knee joint performance, providing insights into power output and muscle coordination.
- **Analysis:**
    - **Inertial Mode:** Focus on the RFD during the push-off phase and the athlete's ability to decelerate effectively during running. This is crucial for identifying inefficiencies or imbalances that could limit speed or increase the risk of injury.
    - **Isokinetic Mode:** Analyze the coordination between the lower limb segments during knee extension and flexion, especially under varying loads. A study conducted by Sánchez-Sánchez et al. (2021) have highlighted the importance of this assessment in understanding the knee's response to different training and rehabilitation stimuli.

- **Application:**
  The insights gained from these assessments can be used to design targeted interventions that improve running mechanics, enhance knee stability, and reduce injury risk. For example, if the data reveals imbalances between the quadriceps and hamstrings, specific strength training protocols can be implemented to correct these issues. Additionally, in rehabilitation contexts, the FEMD can help tailor programs that progressively restore knee function following injury.

Change of Direction

Change of direction (COD) is a critical skill in many sports, such as basketball, football, and tennis, where rapid and precise body movements are required to outmaneuver opponents and maintain high levels of performance (Barrera-Domínguez et al. 2024a). The ability to change direction effectively is influenced by several factors, including muscle strength, particularly in the lower limbs, and the coordination of muscle actions such as eccentric, isometric, and concentric contractions.

- **Mode:** *Isometric, Isokinetic, and Inertial*
- **Objective:** Assess the strength characteristics required for efficient change of direction, focusing on eccentric, isometric, and concentric muscle actions at varying cutting angles.
- **Protocol:**
  - **Isometric Mode:** Evaluate the isometric strength of the lower limbs during simulated cutting actions by having the athlete hold a static position at critical joint angles, such as a mid-thigh pull position, which simulates the deceleration phase of a COD.
  - **Isokinetic Mode:** Assess both concentric and eccentric strength during controlled angular velocities that replicate the acceleration and deceleration phases of COD. The FEMD can be used to perform squats or lunges at velocities that mimic the demands of different COD angles, such as 45°, 90°, and 180 °.
  - **Inertial Mode:** Utilize the inertial mode to simulate the rapid changes in load experienced during COD, particularly focusing on the athlete's ability to produce force quickly (RFD) during deceleration and reacceleration.
- **Analysis:**
  - **Strength and COD Performance:** Recent studies highlight the varying importance of different muscle actions depending on the COD angle. Concentric strength is most crucial for shallower angles (e.g., 45°), while

eccentric and isometric strengths are more critical at sharper angles (e.g., 90° and 180 °). The study also emphasizes the importance of RFD, particularly during eccentric actions, for effective COD performance across all angles (Barrera-Domínguez et al. 2024b).

  - **Angular-Specific Strength Demands:** For COD actions at 45°, high levels of concentric strength are necessary to maintain speed with minimal ground contact time. In contrast, 90° and 180° COD require greater isometric and eccentric strength due to the need for substantial deceleration and reacceleration forces. The ability to rapidly generate force during these phases is a key determinant of performance.
  - **Muscle Action Coordination:** Effective COD is not solely dependent on the strength of individual muscle actions but also on the coordination between eccentric, isometric, and concentric contractions. For example, during a 180° COD, the ability to decelerate rapidly using eccentric strength, followed by an explosive concentric contraction, is critical for minimizing time spent in the change and maximizing speed out of the turn.

- **Application:**

  - **Targeted Strength Training:** Based on FEMD assessments, design a strength training program that targets the specific muscle actions most relevant to the athlete's sport and COD demands. For example, athletes who require rapid directional changes at acute angles should focus on enhancing their eccentric and isometric strength, particularly in the lower limbs. Incorporating exercises such as eccentric squats and isometric holds at joint angles specific to COD movements can improve performance.
  - **Performance Monitoring:** Regularly monitor the athlete's strength using FEMD to track improvements in COD performance. The data collected can inform adjustments to training loads and focus areas, ensuring that the athlete develops balanced strength across all relevant muscle actions.
  - **Injury Prevention:** Use FEMD data to identify any imbalances between concentric and eccentric strength, which could predispose athletes to injuries during COD. Addressing these imbalances through targeted training can reduce the risk of injuries such as ACL tears, which are common in sports involving frequent directional changes.

Stabilization

Trunk stabilization is essential in a wide range of sports, providing the foundation for efficient movement, force transmission, and injury prevention. The comprehensive evaluation of trunk strength, particularly the stabilization and rotator muscles of the trunk, plays a critical role in enhancing athletic performance and supporting effective rehabilitation strategies.

Practical Evaluation of Trunk Stabilization Using FEMD

- **Mode:** Isometric and Isokinetic
- **Objective:** Assess and enhance trunk stabilization and rotator muscle strength, focusing on core strength dynamics crucial for athletic performance and injury prevention.
- **Protocol:**
    - **Isometric Mode:** Use the FEMD to evaluate static trunk stabilization by having the athlete maintain a stable posture, such as a plank or side plank, while the device measures the force output of the trunk stabilizers. This mode is particularly effective in assessing the endurance and maximum strength of the trunk muscles under sustained loads.
    - **Isokinetic Mode:** Employ the Isokinetic mode to assess the dynamic strength of trunk rotators during controlled rotational movements, such as the horizontal cable woodchop (HCW) and low cable woodchop (LCW) exercises. These exercises mimic sport-specific movements and allow for the assessment of both concentric and eccentric muscle contractions at various speeds.
- **Analysis:**
    - **Trunk Rotator Strength and Reliability:** Recent studies such as those by Rodríguez-Perea et al. (2023a, 2023b) emphasize the importance of reliable assessment methodologies for trunk rotator muscles. These studies demonstrated that the HCW exercise, performed at 0.40 ms^{-1}, is highly reliable for measuring trunk rotator strength. Such findings confirm the FEMD's utility in reliably quantifying trunk rotator strength, making it an invaluable tool for both performance assessment and rehabilitation.
    - **Core Strength and Athletic Performance:** The trunk's role in stabilizing the body and transferring forces is critical in sports, such as tennis, canoe sprinting, and golf, where strong trunk rotators contribute to better speed, paddle force, and swing dynamics. The studies by Rodríguez-Perea et al. (2023c) also highlight the importance of integrating both static and dynamic assessments in training programs.
    - **Injury Prevention and Rehabilitation:** Its suggested that isokinetic training can significantly reduce pain and disability in individuals with low back pain by improving trunk muscle function. This aligns with the broader understanding that robust trunk strength not only enhances performance but also plays a crucial role in injury prevention, particularly in the lower back and lower limbs.

- **Application:**
    - **Targeted Training and Rehabilitation:** Based on the FEMD assessment, design a training program that targets both the stabilization and rotational strength of the trunk. For example, incorporate isometric holds combined with dynamic rotational exercises such as the HCW and LCW to develop both endurance and dynamic power in the trunk muscles. These exercises should be performed at the speeds identified as most reliable, ensuring that the training closely aligns with the demands of the athlete's sport.
    - **Performance Monitoring:** Regularly assess trunk strength using FEMD to monitor improvements and adjust training loads accordingly. The reliability of these assessments allows for precise tracking of an athlete's progress, enabling the optimization of both performance and injury prevention strategies.
    - **Holistic Approach to Core Strength:** Integrate findings from isometric and isokinetic evaluations into a comprehensive core strengthening program. This program should not only focus on trunk rotators but also include exercises that enhance overall core stability, ensuring that athletes maintain a strong, resilient trunk capable of supporting high-performance outputs.

Overhead Throwing

Overhead throwing is a complex and dynamic gesture critical to sports such as handball and baseball, where the ability to generate high velocity and precise throws can significantly influence performance outcomes. The assessment of shoulder strength, particularly internal rotation (IR) strength, is vital for both performance enhancement and injury prevention. Leveraging FEMDs for these assessments provides precise and reliable measurements that can guide targeted training and rehabilitation programs.

Proposed Evaluation

- **Mode:** *Isokinetic and Isometric*
- **Objective:** Assess shoulder rotational strength and its relationship to throwing velocity, with a focus on internal rotation (IR) and external rotation (ER) strength.
- **Protocol:**
    - **Isokinetic Mode:** Utilize the Isokinetic mode to measure concentric and eccentric strength during shoulder internal and external rotations. This mode allows for the control of movement speed, providing consistent resistance throughout the range of motion, which is critical for

evaluating how strength in these movements translates to throwing performance.

- **Isometric Mode:** Apply the Isometric mode to assess the static strength of the shoulder rotators, particularly in positions that mimic the critical phases of the throwing motion. This evaluation provides insights into the muscle's ability to stabilize the shoulder during high-velocity throws.

- **Analysis:**
  - **Shoulder Strength and Throwing Velocity:** Studies such as García-Buendía et al. (2022) and Martínez-García et al. (2020) have highlighted the complex relationship between shoulder strength and throwing velocity suggesting that performance is not solely dependent on one aspect of shoulder strength but rather on the integration of multiple strength factors within the kinetic chain.
  - **Kinetic Chain Integration:** The shoulder's role in overhead throwing is part of a larger kinetic chain that involves the coordination of the entire body to maximize energy transfer and throwing velocity. Identifying key predictors of throwing velocity, such as horizontal abduction, internal rotation strength, and trunk rotation power, is essential for understanding how each segment contributes to overall performance. The integration of these elements ensures that energy is transferred correctly, minimizing losses and maximizing both velocity and accuracy in the throw.
  - **Holistic Strength Development:** The lack of a direct correlation between IR strength and throwing velocity challenges the traditional focus on isolated muscle training. Instead, a holistic approach that considers the interplay of various shoulder movements and their contribution to the kinetic chain is recommended. This approach aligns with the findings from the studies mentioned, advocating for diversified training that strengthens multiple aspects of shoulder function.

- **Application:**
  - **Targeted Training:** Based on the evaluation, develop a training program that not only focuses on increasing IR strength but also incorporates exercises targeting horizontal abduction, external rotation, and overall shoulder stability. For example, incorporating resistance training that simulates the throwing motion at varying speeds can enhance both strength and coordination within the kinetic chain.
  - **Injury Prevention:** Use the FEMD data to identify potential imbalances between IR and ER strength, which could predispose athletes to shoulder injuries, such as rotator cuff tears or impingement. By addressing these imbalances through targeted strengthening exercises, the risk of injury can be mitigated, thereby extending the athlete's career longevity.

- **Performance Enhancement:** Regularly monitor shoulder strength using FEMD to track progress and adjust training loads accordingly. The integration of isokinetic and isometric assessments ensures that the athlete develops balanced shoulder strength that supports both high-velocity throws and the ability to withstand the repetitive stresses of competition.

Practical Application for Sport Performance

To generate your own sport-specific assessments using the FEMD, consider the following steps:

1. Identify the Key Gestures in the Sport: Begin by identifying the critical movements that define success in the athlete's sport. For example, in basketball, key gestures might include jumping for rebounds, quick directional changes, and overhead shooting.
2. Select the Appropriate FEMD Mode: Choose the FEMD mode that best replicates the resistance and movement patterns of these key gestures. For example, use the isotonic mode for jump squats to assess explosive lower-body power or the isokinetic mode to evaluate the shoulder strength required for overhead throws in handball.
3. Customize the Assessment Protocol: Tailor the assessment protocol to the athlete's needs by adjusting parameters such as resistance levels, speed, and range of motion. This customization ensures that the assessment closely mirrors the actual demands of the sport.
4. Record and Analyze Data: Utilize the FEMD's capacity to record force data every millisecond throughout the gesture. Analyze the generated reports to assess variables such as strength, range of motion, power, work, and momentum. Pay particular attention to both average and maximum values, as these provide critical insights into the athlete's performance capabilities and potential areas for improvement.
5. Interpret Results for Practical Application: Use the insights gained from the FEMD assessments to inform training and rehabilitation programs. For instance, if the assessment reveals a deficit in eccentric strength during a specific gesture, integrate targeted eccentric training exercises to address this weakness. Similarly, if the data shows a limited range of motion, incorporate flexibility and mobility exercises into the athlete's routine.

By adhering to these recommendations, derived from both the academic insights provided by the latest research and practical application knowledge, coaches and trainers can harness the full potential of FEMD in developing targeted, effective training and rehabilitation programs. This strategic approach not only enhances athletic performance but also plays a crucial role in injury prevention, marking a significant advancement in sports science and athlete management.

References

Barrera-Domínguez, Francisco J., Bartolomé J. Almagro, and Jorge Molina-López. 2024a. "The Influence of Functional Movement and Strength upon Linear and Change of Direction Speed in Male and Female Basketball Players." *Journal of Human Kinetics* 92: 147–159. https://doi.org/10.5114/jhk/177313.

Barrera-Domínguez, Francisco J., Indya del-Cuerpo, Antonio Riego-Ruiz, Darío Martínez-García, Daniel Jerez-Mayorga, Luís Javier Chirosa-Ríos, and Jorge Molina-López. 2024b. "Strength Characteristics in Faster Change of Direction Basketball Players: A Comparison Across Cutting Angles." *European Journal of Sport Science*. https://doi.org/10.1002/ejsc.12164.

Bencke, Jesper, Derek Curtis, Christina Krogshede, Line Klemmensen Jensen, Thomas Bandholm, and Mette Kreutzfeldt Zebis. 2013. "Biomechanical Evaluation of the Side-Cutting Manoeuvre Associated with ACL Injury in Young Female Handball Players." *Knee Surgery, Sports Traumatology, Arthroscopy* 21 (8): 1876–1881. https://doi.org/10.1007/s00167-012-2199-8.

Bittencourt, N. F. N., W. H. Meeuwisse, L. D. Mendonça, A. Nettel-Aguirre, J. M. Ocarino, and S. T. Fonseca. 2016. "Complex Systems Approach for Sports Injuries: Moving from Risk Factor Identification to Injury Pattern Recognition—Narrative Review and New Concept." *British Journal of Sports Medicine* 50 (21): 1309–1314. https://doi.org/10.1136/bjsports-2015-095850.

Bourne, Matthew N., Ryan G. Timmins, David A. Opar, Tania Pizzari, Joshua D. Ruddy, Casey Sims, Morgan D. Williams, and Anthony J. Shield. 2018. "An Evidence-Based Framework for Strengthening Exercises to Prevent Hamstring Injury." *Sports Medicine* 48 (2): 251–267. https://doi.org/10.1007/s40279-017-0796-x.

Cerda Vega, Enrique, Daniel Jerez-Mayorga, Christian Campos Jara, Iris Guzman-Guzman, Alvaro Reyes Ponce, and Luis Javier Chirosa. 2018. "Validity and Reliability of Evaluating Hip Abductor Strength Using Different Normalization Methods in a Functional Electromechanical Device." *PLoS One* 8 (13): 1–12.

Cools, Ann M., Annelies G. Maenhout, Fran Vanderstukken, Philippe Declève, Fredrik R. Johansson, and Dorien Borms. 2020. "The Challenge of the Sporting Shoulder: From Injury Prevention through Sport-Specific Rehabilitation Toward Return to Play." *Annals of Physical and Rehabilitation Medicine*. https://doi.org/10.1016/j.rehab.2020.03.009.

García-Buendía, G., D. Martínez-García, D. Jerez-Mayorga, M. Gómez-López, I. J. Chirosa-Ríos, and L. J. Chirosa-Ríos. 2022. "Exploration of the Shoulder Internal Rotation's Influence on Throwing Velocity in Handball Players: A Pilot Study." *International Journal of Environmental Research and Public Health* 19 (23). https://doi.org/10.3390/ijerph192315923.

Garcia-Pinillos, Felipe, Jose C. Cámara-Pérez, Víctor M. Soto-Hermoso, and Pedro A. Latorre-Román. 2017. "A High Intensity Interval Training (HIIT)-Based Running Plan Improves Athletic Performance by Improving Muscle Power." *Journal of Strength and Conditioning Research* 31 (1): 146–153. https://doi.org/10.1519/JSC.0000000000001473.

Garcia-Ramos, Amador, Alejandro Perez-Castilla, Francisco Villar-Macias, Pedro Ángel Latorre-Román, Juan A. Parraga, and Felipe Garcia-Pinillos. 2018. "Differences in the One-Repetition Maximum and Load-Velocity Profile between the Flat and Arched Bench Press in Competitive Powerlifters." *Sports Biomechanics* 20 (3): 261–273. https://doi.org/10.1080/14763141.2018.1544662.

Greig, Matt, and Ben Langley. 2024. "Exploring the Issue of 'Functionality' in Isokinetic Dynamometry." *Research in Sports Medicine* 32 (5): 804–809. https://doi.org/10.1080/15438627.2023.2260521.

Harry, John R., John Krzyszkowski, Katie Harris, Luke Chowning, Ethan Mackey, Chris Bishop, and Leland A. Barker. 2022. "Momentum-Based Load Prescriptions: Applications to Jump Squat Training." *Journal of Strength and Conditioning Research* 36 (9): 2657–2662. https://doi.org/10.1519/JSC.0000000000004294.

Issurin, V. 2010. "New Horizons for the Methodology and Physiology of Training Periodization." Sports Medicine 40 (3): 803–805. https://doi.org/10.2165/11535130-000000000-00000.

Kraemer, William J., and Nicholas A. Ratamess. 2004. "Fundamentals of Resistance Training: Progression and Exercise Prescription." *Medicine and Science in Sports and Exercise* 36 (4): 674–688. https://doi.org/10.1249/01.MSS.0000121945.36635.61.

López-Rivera, Eva, and Juan José González-Badillo. 2012. "The Effects of Two Maximum Grip Strength Training Methods Using the Same Effort Duration and Different Edge Depth on Grip Endurance in Elite Climbers." *Sports Technology* 5 (3–4): 100–110. https://doi.org/10.1080/19346182.2012.716061.

Martinez-Garcia, Dario, Angela Rodriguez-Perea, Paola Barboza, David Ulloa-Díaz, Daniel Jerez-Mayorga, Ignacio Chirosa, and Luis Javier Chirosa Ríos. 2020. "Reliability of a Standing Isokinetic Shoulder Rotators Strength Test Using a Functional Electromechanical Dynamometer: Effects of Velocity." *PeerJ* 8 (October). https://doi.org/10.7717/PEERJ.9951/SUPP-2.

Ramirez-Campillo, Rodrigo, Cristian Alvarez, Antonio Garcia-Hermoso, Justin W. L. Keogh, Felipe Garcia-Pinillos, Lucas A. Pereira, and Irineu Loturco. 2020. "Effects of Jump Training on Jumping Performance of Handball Players: A Systematic Review and Meta-Analysis." *International Journal of Sports Science & Coaching* 15 (4): 1–18.

Reyes-Ferrada, W., L. Chirosa-Ríos, D. Martinez-Garcia, Á. Rodríguez-Perea, and D. Jerez-Mayorga. 2022. "Reliability of Trunk Strength Measurements with an Isokinetic Dynamometer in Non-Specific Low Back Pain Patients: A Systematic Review." *Journal of Back and Musculoskeletal Rehabilitation* 35 (5). https://doi.org/10.3233/BMR-210261.

Reyes-Ferrada, W., L. Chirosa-Ríos, I. Chirosa-Ríos, D. Martínez-García, P. Barboza-Gonzalez, D. Ulloa-Díaz, D. Jerez-Mayorga, and Á. Rodríguez-Perea. 2021. "A New Reliable Device to Assess Trunk Extensors Strength." *Acta of Bioengineering and Biomechanics* 24 (1). https://doi.org/10.37190/ABB-01965-2021-05.

Rodriguez-Perea, Ángela, D. Jerez-Mayorga, Amador García-Ramos, Dario Martínez-García, and Luis J. Chirosa-Ríos. 2021. "Reliability and

Concurrent Validity of a Functional Electromechanical Dynamometer Device for the Assessment of Movement Velocity." *Proceedings of the Institution of Mechanical Engineers, Part P: Journal of Sports Engineering and Technology* (January). https://doi.org/10.1177/17543371209848 83.

Rodríguez-Perea, Angela, Daniel Jerez-Mayorga, María Dolores Morenas-Aguilar, Darío Martínez-García, Ignacio Jesús Chirosa-Ríos, Luis Javier Chirosa-Ríos, and Waleska Reyes-Ferrada. 2023a. "Influence of Sex and Dominant Side on the Reliability of Two Trunk Rotator Exercises." *Applied Sciences* 13 (4): 2441. https://doi.org/10.3390/APP13042441.

Rodríguez-Perea, Angela, M. D. Morenas Aguilar, Raquel Escobar-Molina, Darío Martínez-García, Ignacio Chirosa-Ríos, Daniel Jerez-Mayorga, Luis Chirosa-Ríos, Danica Janicijevic, and Waleska Reyes-Ferrada. 2023b. "Strength Assessment of Trunk Rotator Muscles: A Multicenter Reliability Study." *Healthcare (Switzerland)* 11 (16). https://doi.org/10.3390/healthcare11162331.

Rodríguez-Perea, Ángela, Waleska Reyes-Ferrada, Daniel Jerez-Mayorga, Luis Chirosa Ríos, Roland Van den Tillar, Ignacio Chirosa Ríos, and Dario Martínez-García. 2023c. "Core Training and Performance: A Systematic Review with Meta-Analysis." *Biology of Sport* 40 (4): 975–992. https://doi.org/10.5114/BIOLSPORT.2023.123319.

Ruiz-Alias, Santiago A., Alejandro Pérez-Castilla, Diego Jaén-Carrillo, and Felipe García-Pinillos. 2024. "Order Effect of an 8-Week Concurrent Training Program on the Maximal Fat Oxidation." *Sport Sciences for Health*. https://doi.org/10.1007/s11332-024-01222-8.

Sánchez-Sánchez, Antonio Jesús, Luis Javier Chirosa-Ríos, Ignacio Jesús Chirosa-Ríos, Agustín José García-Vega, and Daniel Jerez-Mayorga. 2021. "Test-Retest Reliability of a Functional Electromechanical Dynamometer on Swing Eccentric Hamstring Exercise Measures in Soccer Players." *PeerJ* 9: e11743. https://doi.org/10.7717/peerj.11743.

Turner, Anthony N., Ben Jones, Perry Stewart, Chris Bishop, Nimai Parmar, Shyam Chavda, and Paul Read. 2019. "Total Score of Athleticism: Holistic Athlete Profiling to Enhance Decision-Making." *Strength and Conditioning Journal* 41 (6): 91–101. https://doi.org/10.1519/SSC.0000000000000506.

Wagner, H., J. Pfusterschmied, M. Tilp, J. Landlinger, S. P. von Duvillard, and E. Müller. 2012. "Upper-Body Kinematics in Team-Handball Throw, Tennis Serve, and Volleyball Spike." *Scandinavian Journal of Medicine and Science in Sports* 24 (2): 345–354. https://doi.org/10.1111/j.1600-0838.2012.01503.x.

7 Training Proposal to Improve Strength in Sports Tasks

Ángela Rodríguez-Perea, Ignacio J. Chirosa Rios, and Álvaro Huerta Ojeda

Introduction

Strength training is the main axis of improvement in sports movements, in terms of both performance and health. Strength enhancement in sports performance can involve various variables, such as increasing maximum strength, the rate of force production, and power. Numerous training methods for strength development. Owing to technological advancements, functional electromechanical dynamometers have been proposed as devices that can operate in different training modes. This device features seven training modes, which are divided into isometric and dynamic (Table 7.1).

Additionally, to improve strength in sports tasks, a multifaceted training approach is recommended, integrating various strength training methodologies tailored to the specific demands of the sport and the athlete's condition.

The FEMD allows coaches to use different training methods within the same session, offering them the opportunity to create general exercises or exercises like sports tasks.

The timing of the season and the athlete's condition will determine the training method. Moreover, this chapter will develop different training proposals that can be used to enhance athletic performance, such as post-activation potentiation, cluster method, and training based on velocity, strength, or power.

Functional Electromechanical Dynamometer Modes

Isometric

This type of training is characterized by maintaining muscle tension without varying the length of the muscle (isometric contractions). Unlike dynamic movements, the goal here is to develop the ability to generate and maintain force in a specific position for a prolonged period. One of the highlights of the isometric tonic mode is the ability to adjust the duration of the contraction and the applied load. This allows for a highly specific approach where intensity and maintenance time are adapted to the demands of each sporting discipline.

DOI: 10.4324/9781003425182-9

Table 7.1 FEMD modes

Mode	*Icon*	*Type*	*Specific variables*	*Common variables*
Isometric	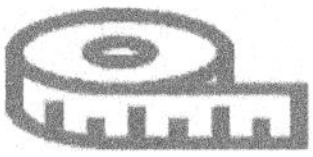	Isometric	Without movement	Time
Isometric Vibratory	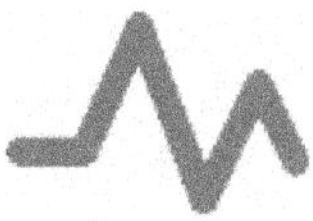	Isometric	Vibration index	Time
Tonic	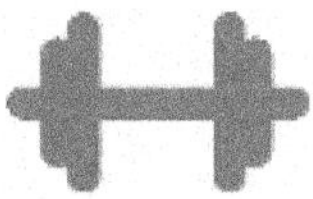	Dynamic	Load at the beginning and end of the concentric phase, and at the beginning and end of the eccentric phase.	Range of movement
Kinetic	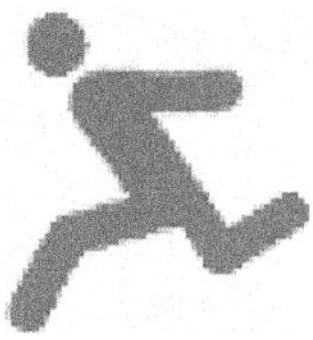	Dynamic	Velocity at the beginning and end of the concentric phase, and at the beginning and end of the eccentric phase.	Range of movement
Elastic	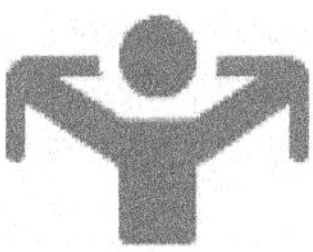	Dynamic	Elastic constant	Range of movement
Inertial	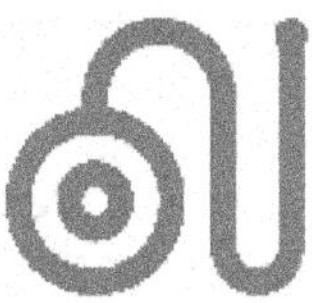	Dynamic	Inertial mass	Range of movement
Conic	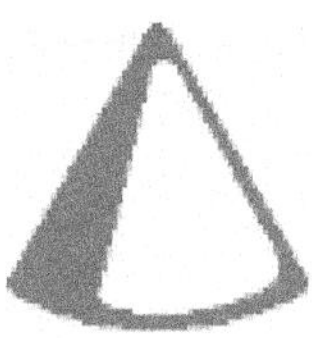	Dynamic	Inertial mass and cone height	Range of movement

The isometric mode is mainly applied in situations where stability and sustained muscular endurance are critical, such as in contact sports (judo, wrestling), where maintaining specific positions under tension is crucial, disciplines that require balance and control, such as gymnastics or yoga, or strength movements in sports, such as cycling or skiing, where a firm posture is needed for a prolonged period of time.

Isometric Vibratory

The use of isometric strength training with vibration represents an advanced approach to enhance muscle performance. This method combines isometric exercises with vibration rate modulation, which allows for additional stimulation and increased muscle activation. The induced vibrations enhance the neuromuscular response, maximizing contraction and isometric training efficiency. The exercises were performed while the rope was held static while it vibrated at a specific frequency. The vibrations generate micro-oscillations that force the muscles to contract reflexively, thereby increasing muscle activation.

Tonic

In tonic mode, the primary adjustable parameter is the load, allowing for the adjustment of the weight to be overcome during different phases as well as at the beginning and end of the movement. If the load is constant, it is referred to as isotonic exercise, whereas if the load increases or decreases, it is referred to as pleotonic exercise. The tonic mode configuration panel is like the kinetic mode configuration panel, with the only difference being that the execution velocity parameter is replaced by the load parameter.

The tonic mode emphasizes maintaining muscle tension and endurance over extended periods. This mode is particularly relevant for sports tasks that demand prolonged force production, stability, and muscle control. The sustained contraction of muscles, especially under varying conditions, is critical in activities where the goal is to resist fatigue while maintaining effective and controlled movement. This mode reproduces a training approach that is performed with external loads. In FEMD, it is possible to know the velocity at which the exercise is being performed as well as the power achieved in each repetition of both the concentric and eccentric phases.

The key to tonic mode training lies in the balance between muscle endurance and controlled strength output. As opposed to velocity-focused approaches, where speed impacts force production, tonic mode training prioritizes maintaining force even as fatigue sets in. The longer the muscle can sustain force, the better the capacity to perform in sports tasks requiring prolonged engagement, such as long-distance running, prolonged defensive positions, or continuous cycling. This mode allows you to adjust the load, the number of repetitions or duration and rest intervals, and can be adapted to meet different performance and rehabilitation goals. For example, in rehabilitation settings, slow, controlled movements in tonic conditions help to restore strength while minimizing the risk of injury. In performance settings, it is applied to improve an athlete's ability to resist fatigue and maintain high levels of control during prolonged efforts.

Kinetic

The execution velocity of movement is a key component in movement dynamics, particularly in sports and activities that require precision and power. The ability to adjust velocity during different phases of a movement, such as the concentric and eccentric phases, is crucial for optimizing force production.

This mode replicates a training based on the execution velocity of the movement, allowing for the adjustment of velocity in different phases as well as at the start and end of the movement. The higher the velocity, the lower the capacity to produce force. Movements are classified based on speed into three main categories:

- Isokinetic Exercises: In these exercises, the execution velocity is constant throughout the entire range of motion. This is achieved using a maintain a preset velocity, allowing for precise evaluation of maximum force at each point in the range of motion. The constant velocity ensures uniform resistance, which is useful for measuring force without the variations introduced by other factors.
- Ascending Pleokinetic Exercises: In this mode, the execution velocity progressively increases throughout the concentric or eccentric phase of the movement. This type of exercise simulates situations where explosiveness is crucial, such as in jumps or throws. However, as velocity increases, the capacity to produce force decreases due to the reduced time available to generate muscular tension.
- Descending Pleokinetic Exercises: In this mode, the velocity progressively decreases, allowing for greater force production toward the end of the range of motion. This strategy is useful in activities requiring precise control during deceleration, such as in landings or deacceleration.

This is consistent with the force-velocity relationship, where a higher speed of muscle contraction is associated with a lower capacity to generate force. Isokinetic exercises allow for constant force production, while pleokinetic exercises provide variability in workload depending on the phase of the movement. Adjusting velocity during the different phases of movement is essential for designing specific training programs that align with the goals of the athlete or patient. Isokinetic exercises are ideal for measuring force capacity under controlled conditions, whereas pleokinetic exercises are more representative of real-life competition or physical activity situations, where speed and force dynamically vary.

This mode can be applied to the design of training routines that optimize force production based on the desired execution speed, providing a personalized approach to improving athletic performance and muscle rehabilitation.

Elastic

Elastic mode replicates the behavior and effects of elastic band training, allowing for variation in the resistance or 'hardness' of the band. This approach is useful for working on muscular strength and endurance through progressive resistance, where the load increases as the band is stretched. The adaptability and versatility of this mode allows for targeted and personalized training. The characteristics of the elastic mode are variable resistance as in this mode, the resistance increases as the range of motion progresses, mimicking the progressive tension of elastic bands. This is useful for movements that require a gradual increase in force. In addition, this simulation allows the resistance to be adjusted according to the 'hardness' of the elastic band, which is determined by the elastic constant in the FEMD. The bands can vary from light to hard (elastic constant), offering multiple load levels to suit training or rehabilitation needs.

The elastic mode is an excellent tool to simulate training with elastic bands, offering an adjustable experience that improves strength, endurance and stability. Its versatility allows its application in multiple contexts, from functional training to rehabilitation, providing a personalized and effective approach to achieve each athlete's goals.

Inertial

The inertial mode is based on the simulation of training with inertial devices, such as Yo-Yo type devices. In this mode, the FEMD allows the adjustment of the inertial mass of the disc. This type of training is highly effective for developing strength in both the concentric and eccentric phases of a movement, where the eccentric resistance is proportional to the force generated in the concentric phase. This mode is especially useful for improving power, deceleration capacity, and injury prevention. In addition, the resistance is not fixed but depends on the energy applied in each repetition. The more force applied in the concentric phase, the greater the resistance in the eccentric phase, forcing the muscle to work hard to control the movement.

Conic

The conic mode simulates training with inertial cone devices, where the force required to manipulate the velocity of the exercise does not depend on a fixed weight, but on the inertia generated by the applied force itself. In this type of training, the greater the force exerted in the concentric phase, the greater the resistance to be controlled in the eccentric phase. This approach is excellent for developing strength, power and eccentric control, replicating the dynamic demands found in most sports. The cone mode in FEMD training offers the possibility to adjust both the weight of the cone and its height, allowing you to customize the intensity and smoothness of the exercise. This adjustment is essential to adapt the training to different fitness levels and specific goals. The higher the height of the cone, the smoother the movement, and the lower the height, the greater the resistance and demand. By adjusting the weight of the cone, the inertia during the exercise is modulated. Heavier cones generate greater resistance, increasing the load during the eccentric phase, as the energy generated in the concentric phase translates into a greater demand for control when returning.

The height of the cone influences the smoothness of the movement. The higher the height, the longer the rope travels, making the exercise more fluid and with less abrupt resistance. This approach is particularly beneficial for beginners, rehabilitation programs, or training scenarios where a more controlled and gradual progression of the load is desired.

Unlike traditional systems that rely on weights, in taper mode the resistance is determined by the velocity and force applied by the user. The more explosive the concentric phase, the greater the eccentric load generated. There is a direct transfer to sporting performance as the taper pattern replicates real sporting situations where the ability to generate and control force is crucial, such as in changes of direction, jumps and explosive movements. As in the inertial mode the eccentric load is proportional, offering a constant challenge, as the resistance in the eccentric phase is directly proportional to the energy generated in the concentric phase, improving both strength and muscle control.

Training Proposals

Use of Functional Electromechanical Dynamometer to Generate Post-activation Performance Enhancement

Post-activation performance enhancement (PAPE) corresponds to a widely used methodology to transiently increase muscular power (Blazevich and Babault 2019; Prieske et al. 2020). Specifically, PAPE is an increase in maximal isometric or dynamic force, power, and/or movement velocity following muscular activation (Prieske et al. 2020). The description of PAPE establishes three phases: Phase (1) assessment of an unpotentiated physical capacity or motor gesture; Phase (2) application of a stimulus triggering an increase in maximal isometric or dynamic force, power, and/or movement velocity; and Phase (3) reassessment of the physical capacity or motor gesture measured in Phase 1 (Figure 7.1).

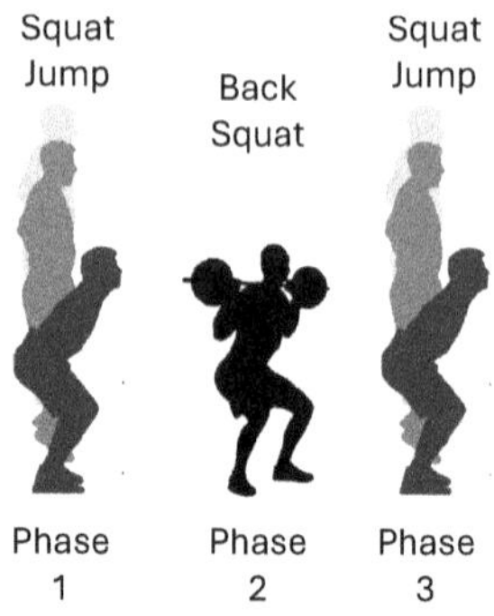

Figure 7.1 Phases 1–3 to obtain PAPE.

In practical terms, it is expected that the level of maximal isometric or dynamic force, power, and/or movement velocity in Phase 3 of the PAPE cycle increases compared to Phase 1. (Ojeda, Ríos, Barrilao, Ríos, et al. 2016). Based on this sequence, Figure 7.1 illustrates an unpotentiated squat jump test in Phase 1. Following this, Phase 2 depicts a back squat aimed at inducing muscular activation, a phase also described in the literature as pre-activation. (Martínez-García et al. 2021). This phase serves the purpose of phosphorylating the light chains of myosin, increasing the recruitment of higher-order motor units, and inducing changes in the pennation angle (Sale 2004; Tillin and Bishop 2009). In the example of Figure 7.1, a back squat is described as pre-activation. Finally, in Phase 3, the exercise from Phase 1 is re-evaluated, in this example, a potentiated squat jump test. It is important to mention that Phase 2 is not conditioned to the back squat exercise, and any exercise involving specific muscle groups can generate PAPE (Soria-Gila et al. 2015; Ojeda, Ríos, Barrilao, Ríos, et al. 2016; Pagaduan and Pojskic 2020). Indeed, up to the development of this chapter, new forms of pre-activation are still being tested (Huerta Ojeda et al. 2023), including complex training (Pagaduan and Pojskic 2020) and contrast training (Talpey, Young, and Saunders 2014), as well as pre-activation with variable resistance (VR) (Huerta Ojeda et al. 2023).

Another important consideration during the application of PAPE is the rest time between pre-activation and Phase 3. In this regard, the existing scientific information is extensive and varied, as PAPE has been evidenced to occur in the first few seconds after pre-activation (Ojeda, Ríos, Barrilao, and Serrano 2016) up to 20 minutes after Phase 2 (Maroto-Izquierdo, Bautista, and Rivera 2020). However, there is no consensus in practice regarding the pause time between these two phases. Despite this, in most research, it has been observed that performance deteriorates within 30 seconds after pre-activation (Martínez-García et al. 2021; Maroto-Izquierdo, Bautista, and Rivera 2020). Beyond this time, with greater certainty after three minutes of rest, PAPE can be achieved (Maroto-Izquierdo et al., 2020).

Variable Resistance

VR has demonstrated good results in developing muscular strength and power (Soria-Gila et al. 2015; Ojeda, Ríos, Barrilao, Ríos, et al. 2016; Pagaduan and Pojskic 2020), with its main characteristic being the variation of intensity within the training load (Thapa et al. 2021). Despite the specificity of the concept, VR can be subclassified into three modalities:

a) Intra-session variable resistance (I-SVR), characterized by the modification of loads between different sets within a training session.
b) Intra-series variable resistance (I-sVR), characterized by the variation of intensities within each set (the intensity of each repetition can be set in percentages of one-repetition maximum [% of 1RM] or in execution velocity [ms^{-1}]).
c) Intra-repetition variable resistance (I-RVR), characterized by variation of resistance during each repetition; in these cases, the use of elastic bands, chains, or functional electromechanical dynamometer is common, allowing for variation in load intensity during each repetition (Mascarin et al. 2017; Wallace, Bergstrom, and Butterfield 2018; Ojeda, Ríos, Barrilao, Ríos, et al. 2016) (Figure 7.2).

From a physiological perspective, VR increases the excitability of motor neurons (Ebben 2002), leading to an increase in phosphorylation of the light chains of myosin, enhanced adenosine triphosphate (ATP) activity, the improved contractile capacity of muscle fibers, and increased motor recruitment, primarily of type II muscle fibers (Sale 2004; Tillin and Bishop 2009).

Use of VR via a Functional Electromechanical Dynamometer to Generate PAPE

Among other purposes, VR has been utilized as a methodology to enhance athletic performance through increased maximal isometric or dynamic strength, power, and/or movement velocity (PAPE) (Blazevich and Babault 2019; Prieske et al. 2020). In this context, FEMDs have provided extensive versatility in the use and application of various forms of VR, in terms of both execution possibilities and load quantification (Martínez-García et al. 2021).

I-RVR Through FEMD

The FEMD manufactured by MYOQUALITY SOLUTIONS (Granada, Spain) model M1, in its tonic mode, allows training with different forms of I-RVR, either with increased resistance at the end of the repetition (emulating a resistance band or chain) or with decreased resistance at the end of the repetition (emulating a sports gesture such as a ball throw or kick). Additionally, the device enables programming of load intensity through kilograms or movement

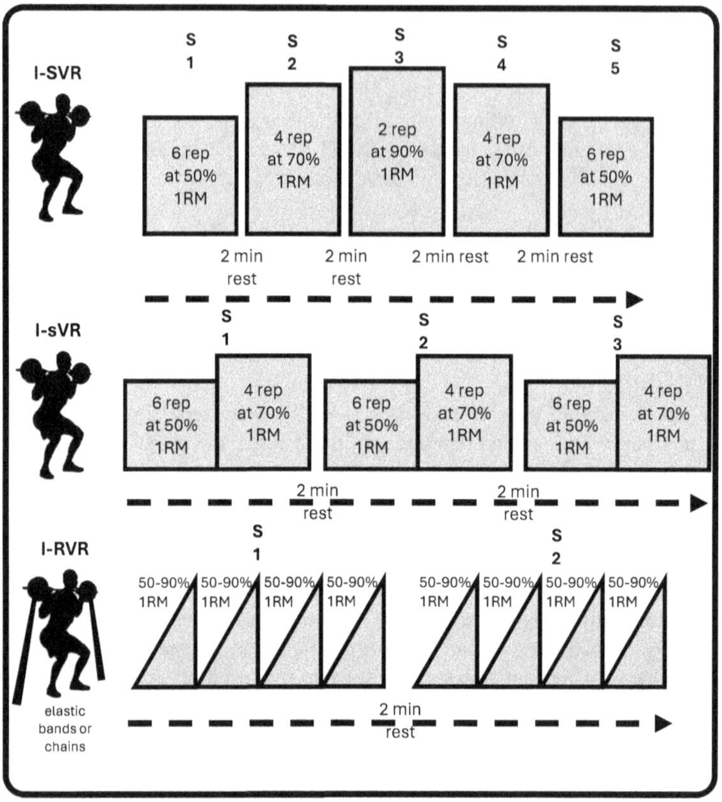

Figure 7.2 Different forms of variable resistance.

velocity (ms^{-1} or kmh^{-1}). In this context, Martínez-García et al. (2021) studied the acute effect of pre-activation with I-RVR, using a FEMD, on overhead throwing velocity in handball players (Martínez-García et al. 2021).

Specifically, pre-activation with VR was used in unilateral bench press (dominant limb) in a standing position, quantifying the load intensity in ms^{-1} (1×5: initial velocity equivalent to 0.6 ms^{-1} and final velocity equivalent to 0.9 ms^{-1}). In individual responses, the analysis showed that 86% of participants increased throwing velocity, concluding that I-RVR generates increases in muscular power, manifested by an increase in overhead throwing velocity in handball players. Other research has reported positive effects (PAPE) through I-RVR (Wyland, Van Dorin, and Reyes 2015; Scott, Ditroilo, and Marshall 2018). However, these studies used resistance bands as I-RVR, making it difficult to replicate the load intensity used in these protocols. Nevertheless, some

FEMDs allow reliable quantification of load intensity, such as Dynasystem in its elastic mode. It is worth noting that these modalities in FEMDs require further exploration.

I-sVR Through FEMD

In its tonic mode, Dynasystem also allows for adjusting loads to create sessions with I-sVR. Specifically, series can be planned and executed with load adjustments in each of the repetitions, either with higher intensity repetitions at the beginning or end of each set (Figure 7.2), emulating sessions where dumbbells are manually loaded and/or unloaded with weight plates during the set. Additionally, the device enables programming of load intensity through kilograms or movement velocity (ms^{-1} or kmh^{-1}).

From practical experience, in an unpublished longitudinal study, we investigated the acute effect of pre-activation with I-sVR, using a FEMD, on overhead throwing velocity in female handball players. Specifically, pre-activation with VR was used in bilateral bench press in a standing position, quantifying the load intensity in ms^{-1} (4 × [1 × 4 at 1.0–1.1 ms^{-1} + 1 × 4 at 0.6–0.7 ms^{-1}], with a three-minute rest interval between sets). Statistical analysis was conducted using repeated measures ANOVA, showing significant differences between the baseline (BL) and the four experimental sets ($P = 0.02$) (Figure 7.3), concluding that I-sVR generates increases in muscular power, manifested in an increase

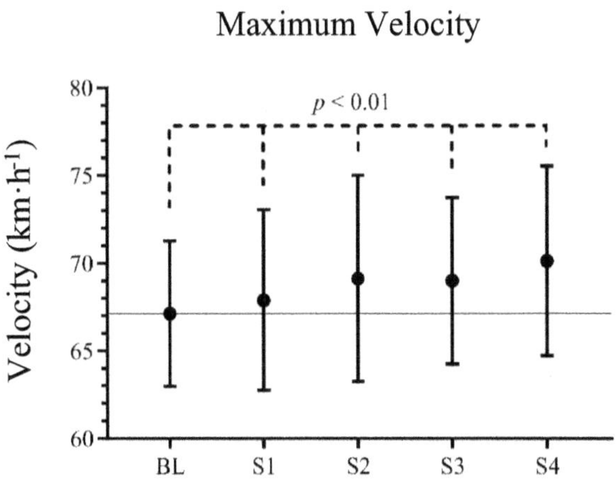

BL = baseline; S1 = set 1; S2 = set 2; S3 = set 3; S4 = set 4;
p = statistical significance

Figure 7.3 Effect of I-sVR on throwing velocity.

in overhead throwing velocity in female handball players. Although this evidence with FEMD is pioneering in quantifying load intensity through I-sVR to trigger PAPE, the tonic modes of these devices require further exploration.

Conclusions and Suggestions

1. PAPE stands as an efficient method for enhancing explosive strength in sports, with ongoing exploration regarding its methodologies.
2. VR, in all its forms, has demonstrated positive effects in triggering PAPE.
3. It is recommended that regardless of the method employed to induce PAPE, coaches and athletes carefully consider training objectives and the magnitude of the effect of different available methodologies (Ng, Chen, and Lum 2020). Furthermore, individual responses to various stimuli should be assessed, as they can vary significantly among athletes (Martínez-García et al. 2021).

These conclusions and suggestions can aid in optimizing training planning and the selection of methods to enhance athletic performance.

Use of Functional Electromechanical Dynamometer in Cluster Sets Configuration

The cluster training method involves incorporating brief rest periods between repetitions within training sets. Due to the rest periods used in this methodology, there may be an increase in substrate availability, which could result in maintaining movement velocity throughout an entire set and training session (Tufano, Brown, and Haff 2017). These set configurations stand out as effective approaches for maintaining mechanical load while simultaneously reducing metabolic and perceptual responses compared to traditional configurations, which involve continuous repetitions (García-Ramos et al. 2020). Following the recommendations of Tufano et al., 2017, the cluster methodology should be used to:

- Ensure the maintenance of velocity and power.
- Increase the total load volume and total work within a session.
- Enhance vertical jump performance.
- Reduce an athlete's Rate of Perceived Exertion.
- Maintain exercise technique and range of motion.
- Incorporate movements where the stretch-shortening cycle plays an important role.
- Acutely reduce cardiovascular stress during strength training.
- Implement post-activation potentiation under strict time constraints.

Cluster sets are effective for improving performance because it allows for greater training volume, and therefore can be considered a beneficial tool when seeking to increase both maximal strength and muscle hypertrophy (García-Ramos et al. 2016; Tufano et al. 2017). Additionally, it has proven to be effective in injury prevention, showing that this methodology reduces the risk of shoulder and knee injuries (Asker et al. 2022).

A recent meta-analysis analyzed optimal training sequences for developing lower body strength, velocity, power and jump height, including cluster training protocols (Marshall et al. 2021). The results showed that peak force was higher in the cluster protocol with a trivial effect [ES: 0.14, 95% CI (−0.21, 0.48), $P =$ 0.44], peak velocity was higher in the cluster protocol with a large positive effect [ES: 1.07, 95% CI (0.58, 1.55), $P <$ 000.1], and peak power was higher in the cluster protocol with a small positive effect [ES: 0.42, 95% CI (0.18, 0.65), $P = 0.0005$]. The results showed that peak force was higher in the cluster protocol with a trivial effect [ES: 0.14, 95% CI (−0.21, 0.48), $P = 0.44$], peak velocity was higher in the cluster protocol with a large positive effect [ES: 1.07, 95% CI (0.58, 1.55), $P < 0.0001$] and peak power was higher in the cluster protocol with a small positive effect [ES: 0.42, 95% CI (0.18, 0.65), $P = 0.0005$].

In addition, useful conclusions for the use of this type of training can be taken from the articles included in this meta-analysis:

1. Six seconds between repetitions is enough to induce partial recovery during the half squat exercise (García-Ramos et al. 2016).
2. Cluster protocols maintained average propulsive velocity better than traditional squat protocols (González-Hernández et al. 2020).
3. Clusters appear to maintain peak power and peak velocity compared to traditional training during squat jump (Hansen, Cronin, and Newton 2011). For non-elite individuals, the maximum power output of jump squat exercise was approximately 4% greater in a session with cluster sets compared to a session with traditional sets (Koefed et al. 2018).
4. Higher peak velocity occurred during the cluster set when compared with the traditional sets at both intensities during a clean pull (Haff et al. 2003).
5. A cluster-set configuration allows for a higher number of repetitions and improved sustainability of mechanical performance during parallel squat (Iglesias-Soler et al. 2014).

Considering all the benefits that cluster training can provide and the advantages of the FEMD over other evaluation and training modes, an evaluation and training protocol is proposed for sports in which achieving high levels of strength and power is crucial. The FEMD allows determination of the power zone of a specific exercise on an individual basis. This can be done in either the tonic or kinetic modes. In this case, we will explain how to perform an incremental load test to determine the power zone for upper body exercise (unilateral press in a bipedal position) and core exercise (woodchop on a low pulley) using the tonic mode. Before starting the evaluation, the execution position and technique of the exercise should be explained to the athlete.

Instructions for the Unilateral Press Exercise:

1. The foot opposite the executing arm should be positioned forward.
2. Hold the grip with the dominant hand, with the palm facing down.
3. The initial position is with the fist at shoulder height, elbow fully flexed, and forearm parallel to the ground.
4. With a slight knee flexion (<20°), push the elbow to full extension as quickly as possible to reach the maximum point of the range of motion without moving the legs.
5. Attempt to pull the cord as quickly as possible and follow through with the movement as it recoils.
6. Feedback and encouragement will be given to the athlete.

Instructions for the Woodchop Exercise:

1. The feet should be shoulder width apart.
2. Hold the grip with both hands below the hip, with both arms extended.
3. The initial arm position is with the elbows extended, and the grip should be in contact with the athlete's thigh.
4. With slight knee flexion (<20°), the torso is rotated energetically while raising the arms diagonally to the maximum point of the range of motion without moving the legs.
5. Attempt to pull the cord as quickly as possible and follow through with the movement as it recoils.
6. Feedback and encouragement will be given to the athlete.

Additionally, the athlete will be instructed to perform as many repetitions as possible without losing technique or range of motion. After explaining the evaluation procedure, the FEMD was configured for the given exercise. The initial load is set, which can be either the same for all athletes or individualized based on the percentage of body weight or maximal isometric strength. In this case, the protocol will use 30% of the athlete's maximal isometric strength for the exercise, previously evaluated with FEMD in isometric mode in the starting position for 6 seconds. For example, if the athlete exerts a maximal isometric force of 30 kg, incremental evaluation in tonic mode will start with a force of 9 kg.

To evaluate power using the FEMD, an incremental test will be conducted, starting the test with 30% of the maximal isometric strength and increasing by 2–4 kg per repetition. The increment will depend on the body weight of each athlete (<60 kg body weight, 2 kg increment; 60–80 kg body weight,

2 kg increment; <80 kg body weight, 4 kg increment). The FEMD allows for load increments between repetitions via the tonic mode control panel.

Prior to performing the exercises, athletes must become familiar with specific movements. They performed a set of eight repetitions of the exercise with resistance bands, followed by three repetitions in the FEMD group, with 30% of their maximal isometric strength. Once the incremental test has been performed, the power zone is determined. This zone corresponds to the load used during training sessions.

To improve power in a specific exercise, a strength training regimen with a cluster set configuration was proposed. Three sets of 15 repetitions will be performed with a 5-s rest between repetitions. Every five repetitions within a set, a five-second rest will be taken (5 reps + 5" rest + 5 reps + 5" rest). Training will be conducted in tonic mode, focusing on performing the concentric phase at the maximum possible speed with the load that produces the maximum power during the incremental test. The number of exercises performed, as well as the volume, will depend on the stage of the season in which the athlete is undergoing and will be determined by the strength coach or trainer.

Thanks to the FEMD's mechanics, to rest between repetitions, the athlete simply needs to stop exerting force. The FEMD consists of a rope that extends from the device (concentric phase) and recoils (eccentric phase). Therefore, when the athlete does not exert tension, the rope does not extend from the device. Athletes will be instructed that after completing the first five repetitions of the set, they should not exert tension and take a five-second rest before performing five more repetitions at maximum speed, repeating the process to complete the 15 repetitions.

Use of Functional Electromechanical Dynamometer in Velocity-Based Training

VBT has emerged as a powerful tool in resistance training, enabling athletes and coaches to tailor workouts based on the velocity of movement rather than relying solely on traditional methods like percentage-based training. The introduction of devices such as functional electromechanical dynamometers has further enhanced this approach, providing detailed feedback on velocity, force and power, leading to more precise and individualized training programs.

The aim of this section is to explore the integration of VBT, with FEMD, providing a detailed understanding of how to effectively use these tools to optimize resistance training outcomes. To successfully incorporate VBT with FEMD into a training regimen, it is essential to meet the following prerequisites:

1. Technical Mastery: Athletes should possess a solid understanding and execution of the exercises where VBT will be applied. Proper form and technique are paramount to ensuring accurate data collection and minimizing injury risks.

2. Accurate Measurement Tools: The reliability of FEMDs is crucial, as they provide the data that will guide training adjustments. Ensure that the device you use has been validated for accuracy and consistency in measuring both velocity and force.
3. Maximal Intent: Athletes must consistently train with the intent to move the load as quickly as possible during the concentric phase of the movement. This intent is critical for the effectiveness of VBT, as it ensures that the data collected reflects true performance capacity.

The cornerstone of VBT is the load-velocity relationship, which indicates that as the load increases, the velocity of the movement decreases in a predictable manner. This relationship is linear across most of the loading spectrum, typically between 40% and 90% of 1RM. By utilizing FEMDs, this relationship can be accurately plotted, allowing for precise load adjustments based on real-time feedback.

- Linearity: The load-velocity relationship remains linear across a broad range of loads, allowing for accurate predictions of performance and adaptations.
- Stability: Once established, an athlete's load-velocity profile remains relatively stable over time, even with changes in 1RM. This stability enables long-term programming adjustments without the need for frequent re-testing.

Training with VBT, especially when combined with FEMDs, leads to significant physiological adaptations. These include improvements in both neural and structural components of strength:

1. Neural Adaptations: Training with maximal velocity intention enhances the nervous system's ability to generate force quickly, improves intra- and inter-muscular coordination, and reduces co-activation of antagonistic muscles, leading to more efficient movement patterns.
2. Structural Adaptations: VBT also promotes structural adaptations, such as increased muscle fiber contraction speed, which is crucial for explosive movements in athletic performance.

In addition, FEMDs allow for the measurement of various velocity-related metrics, each offering unique insights into the athlete's performance:

1. Mean Velocity: The average speed during the entire concentric phase of the movement.
2. Peak Velocity: The highest speed achieved during the concentric phase, offering insight into the athlete's explosive power.
3. Mean Propulsion Velocity: The average speed during the propulsion phase, excluding the deceleration phase, to better understand force application.
4. Rate of Force Development (RFD): A unique measure provided by FEMDs, indicating the speed at which force is generated, which is particularly relevant for explosive sports.

The use of FEMDs in VBT provides immediate feedback on performance, which has been shown to significantly enhance motivation and drive progress. For instance, a study involving professional rugby players demonstrated that those receiving real-time feedback on their execution speeds saw greater improvements in performance metrics compared to those who did not receive such feedback (Weakley et al. 2019).

Moreover, one of the primary advantages of VBT with FEMDs is the ability to regulate training intensity based on real-time data. This can be achieved through two approaches:

1. Generic Load-Velocity Profiles: These profiles allow for quick adjustments based on averaged relative speeds, making them ideal for beginners.
2. Individualized Load-Velocity Profiles: For more advanced athletes, creating an individualized profile provides greater precision. By conducting an incremental protocol to determine the 1RM and corresponding velocities, athletes can tailor their training loads more accurately to their current capabilities.

Example Protocol:

- Begin with light loads (20% 1RM) and incrementally increase, recording the velocity for each load.
- Use this data to create a linear regression model that maps load to velocity, allowing for precise load prescriptions in future sessions.

VBT with FEMDs also facilitates the regulation of training volume, an essential component in preventing overtraining and optimizing recovery:

1. Percentage of Velocity Loss: Setting a threshold for velocity loss during sets (e.g., stopping when velocity decreases by 20%) can prevent excessive fatigue and ensure the athlete remains within the desired training zone.
2. RM-Velocity Profile: By associating specific velocities with corresponding repetition maximums (e.g., 8RM, 12RM), athletes can more accurately determine when to stop a set based on real-time feedback, ensuring they stay within their target rep range and avoid unnecessary fatigue.

Furthermore, FEMDs represent the latest in training technology, offering a more sophisticated approach compared to traditional linear position transducers or inertial sensors. When selecting an FEMD, consider:

1. Validation: Ensure the device has been validated in non-guided, polyarticular movements to guarantee accuracy.
2. Budget: While FEMDs offer advanced features, they can be more expensive. Weigh the benefits against your budget and training needs.
3. Interface Quality: A user-friendly interface is essential for real-time feedback and long-term data tracking.

In conclusion, the integration of VBT with FEMDs offers a cutting-edge approach to resistance training, providing athletes with the tools needed to optimize performance and reduce the risk of overtraining. While not essential for beginners, advanced lifters and coaches can greatly benefit from the precision and feedback offered by these devices. As technology continues to evolve, the accessibility and functionality of FEMDs will likely improve, making them an invaluable asset in the pursuit of athletic excellence.

Below is a table that can be used as a quick reference for setting training parameters using VBT, helping athletes and coaches to adjust loads and monitor performance to achieve specific training goals (Table 7.2). The "velocity range" (m/s) refers to the average velocity of the bar during the concentric phase of the movement for the given load. "Percentage of 1RM" is the estimated percentage of the athlete's 1RM that corresponds to the given velocity range. And the "velocity loss threshold" is the percentage of velocity loss within a set at which the set should be terminated to avoid excessive fatigue and optimize training outcomes.

In addition, Table 7.3 summarizes the key thresholds and concepts used in VBT, especially with the application of FEMD. This table should provide a clear and concise reference for implementing VBT principles with the use of FEMDs, allowing for smarter, more tailored resistance training programs.

Table 7.2 Brief explanation of the focus and approach for each training objective using VBT principles

Training objective	*Velocity range (m/s)*	*Percentage of 1RM*	*Velocity loss threshold*	*Description*
Maximum Strength	0.15–0.35	85%–100%	20%	Focus on heavy loads with a small velocity loss to avoid excessive fatigue.
Strength-Speed	0.35–0.60	70%–85%	20%	Balancing strength and speed, maintaining moderate velocity with relatively heavy loads.
Speed-Strength	0.60–0.85	50%–70%	10%–15%	Emphasizing speed over strength, with lighter loads moved quickly.
Power Development	0.85–1.10	30%–50%	10%–15%	Focus on developing power, moving lighter loads at high speeds, minimal velocity loss to stay fresh.
Muscular Endurance	>1.10	<30%	>40%	Higher velocity loss allowed to focus on endurance, involving higher repetition volumes.

Table 7.3 Reference for implementing VBT principles with the use of FEMDs

VBT concept	*Description*	*Threshold/target*	*Application/use*
Load-Velocity Profile	A linear relationship between load and velocity.	Establish for each major lift; track progress over time.	Use to estimate 1RM without maximal testing; track improvements by observing shifts in the profile line (upward and to the right indicates progress).
Best Rep Velocity	The fastest velocity achieved in a set.	Track the best rep velocity across multiple sessions.	Compare best rep velocity to a 30-day average to gauge progress and readiness; higher best rep velocity typically indicates readiness for increased intensity.
Velocity Loss (% Fatigue)	The percentage decline in velocity from the fastest to the last rep in a set.	Power training: <10%–15% loss; Strength training: <20% loss.	Monitor to regulate training volume and intensity; stop the set when the desired velocity loss threshold is reached to avoid excessive fatigue.
Minimum Velocity Threshold (MVT)	The final rep velocity where the next rep would be failed.	Individualized per lifter and lift; often slower for experienced lifters.	Use to determine proximity to failure and estimate reps in reserve (RIR); closer to MVT indicates higher fatigue and nearing failure.
Intent to Move	The effort to move the load as quickly as possible.	Maintain high intent in every rep for optimal neural adaptations.	Track velocity to ensure consistent high intent; low velocity despite low load may indicate low intent or fatigue.
Power-Load Profile	A curve showing the relationship between load and power output, with a peak point indicating maximum power.	Typically 30%–70% of 1RM.	Use to determine the optimal load for power training; train at or around the load that produces maximum power output for explosive gains.
Autoregulation with Velocity	Adjusting training based on real-time velocity data.	Green light: >95% of 30-day average; Amber light: <95%.	Adjust sets, reps, or load based on velocity feedback during warm-ups; push harder on "green light" days, ease off on "amber light" days.
Training Zones for Specific Adaptations	Targeting specific adaptations (e.g., power, strength) by training at specific velocities and loads.	Power: Focus on loads at peak power velocity (30%–70% 1RM).	Optimize training by matching load and velocity to desired outcomes (e.g., use dynamic effort with peak power loads for explosive power development).
Velocity Progression	Progressing training based on velocity improvements.	Increase load or reps when velocity targets are consistently met.	Set specific velocity goals (e.g., maintain >0.4 m/s with a given load) and progress training load only when these targets are achieved consistently.

Load-Velocity Profile: It is a fundamental tool in VBT, allowing for precise adjustments in training load based on observed velocities.

Best Repetition Velocity: It helps in monitoring peak performance within a set, offering a clear metric to track improvements.

Velocity Loss: It is a practical method to regulate fatigue within sets and maintain training quality.

Minimum Velocity Threshold (MVT): It provides insight into how close an athlete is to failure, useful for programming and adjusting effort.

Intent to Move: It ensures that athletes are putting maximal effort into every rep, crucial for optimizing neural adaptations.

Power-Load Profile: It aids in selecting the optimal load for power development, enhancing training specificity.

Autoregulation with Velocity: It allows for real-time adjustments to training plans, making sessions more responsive to an athlete's current state.

Training Zones: These are less about strict velocity ranges and more about using velocity data to optimize specific training outcomes.

Velocity Progression: It encourages progression based on actual improvements in velocity, ensuring that increases in load are justified by performance gains.

References

Asker, Martin, Martin Hägglund, Markus Waldén, Henrik Källberg, and Eva Skillgate. 2022. "The Effect of Shoulder and Knee Exercise Programmes on the Risk of Shoulder and Knee Injuries in Adolescent Elite Handball Players: A Three-Armed Cluster Randomised Controlled Trial." *Sports Medicine-Open* 8 (1). https://doi.org/10.1186/S40798-022-00478-Z.

Blazevich, Anthony J., and Nicolas Babault. 2019. "Post-Activation Potentiation versus Post-Activation Performance Enhancement in Humans: Historical Perspective, Underlying Mechanisms, and Current Issues." *Frontiers in Physiology* 10 (November): 1359. https://doi.org/10.3389/fphys.2019.01359.

Ebben, William P. 2002. "Complex Training: A Brief Review." *Journal of Sports Science and Medicine* 1: 42–46. www.jssm.org.

García-Ramos, Amador, Jorge M. González-Hernández, Ezequiel Baños-Pelegrín, Adrián Castaño-Zambudio, Fernando Capelo-Ramírez, Daniel Boullosa, G. Gregory Haff, and Pedro Jiménez-Reyes. 2020. "Mechanical and Metabolic Responses to Traditional and Cluster Set Configurations in the Bench Press Exercise." *Journal of Strength and Conditioning Research* 34 (3): 663–70. https://doi.org/10.1519/JSC.0000000000002301.

García-Ramos, Amador, Vicente Nebot, Paulino Padial, Teresa Valverde-Esteve, Ana Pablos-Monzó, and Belén Feriche. 2016. "Effects of Short Inter-Repetition Rest Periods on Power Output Losses during the Half Squat Exercise." *Isokinetics and Exercise Science* 24 (4): 323–30. https://doi.org/10.3233/IES-160634.

González-Hernández, Jorge M., Amador García-Ramos, Adrián Castaño-Zambudio, Fernando Capelo-Ramírez, Gonzalo Marquez, Daniel Boullosa, and Pedro Jiménez-Reyes. 2020. "Mechanical, Metabolic, and Perceptual Acute Responses to Different Set Configurations in Full Squat." *Journal of Strength and Conditioning Research* 34 (6): 1581–90. https://doi.org/10.1519/JSC.0000000000002117.

Haff, G. Gregory, Adrian Whitley, Lora B. Mccoy, Harold S. O'Bryant, J. Lon Kilgore, Erin E. Haff, Kyle Pierce, et al. 2003. "Effects of Different Set Configurations on Barbell Velocity and Displacement during a Clean Pull." *The Journal of Strength & Conditioning Research* 17 (1): 95–103. https://journals.lww.com/nsca-jscr/abstract/2003/020 000/000effects_of_different_set_configurations_on_barbell.16.aspx.

Hansen, Keir T., John B. Cronin, and Michael J. Newton. 2011. "The Effect of Cluster Loading on Force, Velocity, and Power During Ballistic Jump Squat Training." *International Journal of Sports Physiology and Performance* 6 (4): 455–68. https://doi.org/10.1123/IJSPP.6.4.455.

Huerta Ojeda, Álvaro, Claudio Cifuentes Zapata, Guillermo Barahona-Fuentes, María-Mercedes Yeomans-Cabrera, and Luis Javier Chirosa-Ríos. 2023. "Variable Resistance-An Efficient Method to Generate Muscle Potentiation: A Systematic Review and Meta-Analysis." *International Journal of Environmental Research and Public Health* 20 (5): 4316. https://doi.org/10.3390/ijerph20054316.

Iglesias-Soler, Eliseo, Eduardo Carballeira, Tania Sánchez-Otero, Xian Mayo, and Miguel Fernández-Del-Olmo. 2014. "Performance of Maximum Number of Repetitions with Cluster-Set Configuration." *International Journal of Sports Physiology and Performance* 9 (4): 637–42. https://doi.org/10.1123/IJSPP.2013-0246.

Koefed, Nikolaj, Mads Lerche, Bjorn K. Jensen, Pia Kjaer, Sebastian Dam, Rasmus Horslev, and Ernst A. Hansen. 2018. "Peak Power Output in Loaded Jump Squat Exercise Is Affected by Set Structure." *International Journal of Exercise Science* 11 (1): 776. https://doi.org/10.70252/QNBF7275

Maroto-Izquierdo, Sergio, Iker J. Bautista, and Fernando Martín Rivera. 2020. "Post-Activation Performance Enhancement (PAPE) after a Single Bout of High-Intensity Flywheel Resistance Training." *Biology of Sport* 37 (4): 343–50. https://doi.org/10.5114/biolsport.2020.96318.

Marshall, James, Chris Bishop, Anthony Turner, and G. Gregory Haff. 2021. "Optimal Training Sequences to Develop Lower Body Force, Velocity, Power, and Jump Height: A Systematic Review with Meta-Analysis." *Sports Medicine (Auckland, N.Z.)* 51 (6): 1245–71. https://doi.org/10.1007/S40279-021-01430-Z.

Martínez-García, Darío, Ángela Rodríguez-Perea, Álvaro Huerta-Ojeda, Daniel Jerez-Mayorga, Daniel Aguilar-Martínez, Ignacio Chirosa-Rios, Pablo Ruiz-Fuentes, and Luis Javier Chirosa-Rios. 2021. "Effects of Pre-Activation with Variable Intra-Repetition Resistance on Throwing Velocity in Female Handball Players: A Methodological Proposal." *Journal of Human Kinetics* 77 (1): 235–44. https://doi.org/10.2478/hukin-2021-0022.

Mascarin, Naryana Cristina, Claudio Andre Barbosa de Lira, Rodrigo Luiz Vancini, Alberto de Castro Pochini, Antonio Carlos da Silva, and Marilia dos Santos Andrade. 2017. "Strength Training Using Elastic Bands: Improvement of Muscle Power and Throwing Performance in Young Female

Handball Players." *Journal of Sport Rehabilitation* 26 (3): 245–52. https://doi.org/10.1123/jsr.2015-0153.

Ng, Choon Yeow, Siow Ee Chen, and Danny Lum. 2020. "Inducing Postactivation Potentiation with Different Modes of Exercise." *Strength & Conditioning Journal* 42 (2): 63–81. https://doi.org/10.1519/ssc.0000000000000522.

Ojeda, Álvaro Huerta, Luis Chirosa Ríos, Rafael Guisado Barrilao, Ignacio Chirosa Ríos, and Pablo Cáceres Serrano. 2016. "Effect of Post-Activation Potentiation in Athletics: A Systematic Review." *Revista Archivos de Medicina Del Deporte* 33 (5): 338–45.

Ojeda, Álvaro Huerta, Luis Chirosa Ríos, Rafael Guisado Barrilao, and Pablo Cáceres Serrano. 2016. "Acute Effect of a Complex Training Protocol of Back Squats on 30-m Sprint Times of Elite Male Military Athletes." *Journal of Physical Therapy Science* 28 (3): 752–56. https://doi.org/10.1589/jpts.28.752.

Pagaduan, J., and H. Pojskic. 2020. "A Meta-Analysis on the Effect of Complex Training on Vertical Jump Performance." *Journal of Human Kinetics* 71 (1): 255–65. https://doi.org/10.2478/hukin-2019-0087.

Prieske, Olaf, Martin Behrens, Helmi Chaabene, Urs Granacher, and Nicola A Maffiuletti. 2020. "Time to Differentiate Postactivation 'Potentiation' from 'Performance Enhancement' in the Strength and Conditioning Community." *Sports Medicine* 50 (9): 1559–65. https://doi.org/10.1007/s40279-020-01300-0.

Sale, D. 2004. "Postactivation Potentiation: Role in Performance." *British Journal of Sports Medicine* 38 (4): 386–87. https://doi.org/10.1136/bjsm.2002.003392.

Scott, David J., Massimiliano Ditroilo, and Phil Marshall. 2018. "Effect of Accommodating Resistance on the Postactivation Potentiation Response in Rugby League Players." *Journal of Strength and Conditioning Research* 32 (9): 2510–20. https://doi.org/10.1519/JSC.0000000000002464.

Soria-Gila, Miguel, Ignacio Chirosa, Iker Bautista, Salvador Baena, and Luis Chirosa. 2015. "Effects of Variable Resistance Training on Maximal Strength: A Meta-Analysis." *Journal of Strength and Conditioning Research* 29 (11): 3260–70.

Talpey, S W, W B Young, and N Saunders. 2014. "The Acute Effects of Conventional, Complex, and Contrast Protocols on Lower-Body Power." *Journal of Strength and Conditioning Research* 28 (2): 361–66. https://doi.org/10.1519/JSC.0b013e318299a68b.

Thapa, Rohit K., Danny Lum, Jason Moran, and Rodrigo Ramirez-Campillo. 2021. "Effects of Complex Training on Sprint, Jump, and Change of Direction Ability of Soccer Players: A Systematic Review and Meta-Analysis." *Frontiers in Psychology* 11: 1–15. https://doi.org/10.3389/fpsyg.2020.627869.

Tillin, Neale, and David J Bishop. 2009. "Factors Modulating Post-Activation Potentiation and Its Effect on Performance of Subsequent Explosive Activities." *Sports Medicine* 39 (2): 147–66.

Tufano, James J., Lee E. Brown, and G. Gregory Haff. 2017. "Theoretical and Practical Aspects of Different Cluster Set Structures: A Systematic Review." *Journal of Strength and Conditioning Research* 31 (3): 848–67. https://doi.org/10.1519/JSC.0000000000001581.

Wallace, Brian J., Haley C. Bergstrom, and Timothy A. Butterfield. 2018. "Muscular Bases and Mechanisms of Variable Resistance Training Efficacy." *International Journal of Sports Science and Coaching* 13 (6): 1177–88. https://doi.org/10.1177/1747954118810240.

Weakley, Jonathon, Kevin Till, John Sampson, Harry Banyard, Cedric Leduc, Kyle Wilson, Greg Roe, and Ben Jones. 2019. "The Effects of Augmented Feedback on Sprint, Jump, and Strength Adaptations in Rugby Union Players After a 4-Week Training Program." *International Journal of Sports Physiology and Performance* 14 (9): 1205–11. https://doi.org/10.1123/IJSPP.2018-0523.

Wyland, Timothy P., Joshua D Van Dorin, and G Francis Cisco Reyes. 2015. "Postactivation Potentation Effects from Accommodating Resistance Combined with Heavy Back Squats on Short Sprint Performance." *Journal of Strength and Conditioning Research* 29 (11): 3115–23. https://doi.org/10.1519/jsc.0000000000000991.

Section 3

Strength Assessment for Health and Well-Being

8 Relevant Variables in the Assessment of Strength in Health

Daniel Jiménez-Lupión, Daniel Jerez-Mayorga, and Pedro Delgado-Floody

Global Aging Trends and Its Impact on Population Health

The 20th century and the first two decades of the 21st century have witnessed a remarkable rise in global life expectancy. In numerous countries, particularly in Europe and Asia, life expectancy now exceeds 80 years (United Nations, 2019). As a result, the population of elderly individuals has grown substantially. According to World Health Organization (WHO) estimates, the number of people over the age of 60 currently exceeds one billion and is projected to reach two billion by 2050 (World Health Organization, 2015). In this context, it is crucial to establish specific objectives and action plans to promote healthy aging within the population. Healthy aging is defined as the process of developing and maintaining functional capabilities that support well-being in later life. According to the WHO, functional ability includes a range of attributes that enable individuals to engage in valued activities, such as mobility, relationship building and maintenance, self-sufficiency, continuous learning and growth, decision-making, and societal contribution, regardless of chronological age (Frontera, 2022).

Aging has been identified as a major risk factor for the development of chronic non-communicable diseases (World Health Organization, 2014). It is a natural process that affects all living beings and is defined as the natural deterioration of bodily systems over time, including the neuromuscular system (Jakovljevic, 2018). This deterioration leads to a marked decline in muscle mass and, more importantly, muscle function (i.e., strength and power) (Marcell, 2003). Such age-related changes can diminish functional capacity and elevate the risk of disability, falls, and mortality among older adults (Briggs et al., 2016). Furthermore, aging is linked to a state of frailty, defined as increased vulnerability to health issues due to functional decline and decreased reserve capacity (Fried et al., 2001).

The prevalence of frailty is expected to continue rising in the foreseeable future (O'Caoimh et al., 2021). While frailty involves multiple dimensions, including physical, social, and psychological factors, one notable characteristic

DOI: 10.4324/9781003425182-11

linked to physical frailty is sarcopenia. This geriatric syndrome is defined by the loss of skeletal muscle mass, muscle strength and physical performance, due to either aging (primary sarcopenia) or chronic disease (secondary sarcopenia) (Bauer et al., 2019). These age-related changes lead to greater dependence in performing activities of daily living, significantly increasing healthcare costs (Mijnarends et al., 2018) and institutionalization (Martien et al., 2015).

Sarcopenia has traditionally been linked with aging and the elderly; however, it is now understood that the onset of sarcopenia can occur earlier in life and there are numerous factors beyond aging that contribute to its phenotype (Sayer et al., 2008). Moreover, sarcopenia has been identified as both a cause and effect of diabetes mellitus (Hong et al., 2017), linked to cognitive impairment and depression (Chang et al., 2017), and is associated with a heightened risk of ischemic heart disease (Jun et al., 2021). As the global population ages, the incidence of sarcopenia is expected to rise significantly, leading to additional serious adverse consequences and harm (Xie et al., 2020); therefore, the identification and treatment of sarcopenia is of vital importance for health.

Definition and Evolution of the Concept of Sarcopenia

In the past 40 years, two key indicators have been introduced to detect early neuromuscular deterioration in the later stages of life: sarcopenia and dynapenia. In 1988, Irwin H. Rosenberg proposed the concept of "sarcopenia" to describe changes in body composition (reduction in skeletal muscle mass and lean body mass) that affect mobility, independence, and nutritional status (Rosenberg, 1997). The term "sarcopenia," derived from Greek meaning "loss of flesh," was originally proposed to refer to the loss of muscle mass and muscle function related to aging. However, for several decades, it was used solely to refer to the loss of muscle mass, without considering muscle function (Evans, 1995).

Starting in 2000, the term "sarcopenia" evolved to encompass a broader concept that included both the decline in muscle mass and muscle strength (Roubenoff & Hughes, 2000). In 2008, Brian Clark and Todd Manini introduced the concept of "dynapenia," specifically referring to the reduction in muscle strength and power (Clark & Manini, 2008). Subsequently, in 2010, six of the consensus definitions of sarcopenia were updated, incorporating muscle function into the concept (Chen et al., 2014; Cruz-Jentoft et al., 2010; Fielding et al., 2011; Morley et al., 2011; Muscaritoli et al., 2010; Studenski et al., 2014).

The European Working Group on Sarcopenia in Older People (EWGSOP) made a substantial contribution to the operational definition of sarcopenia by underscoring the importance of muscle function and strength, alongside muscle mass. This definition clarified that sarcopenia encompasses both reduced muscle mass and diminished muscle function, which can be evaluated through measurements of muscle strength or physical performance (Cruz-Jentoft et al.,

Table 8.1 Definitions of sarcopenia by EWGSOP2 and AWGS-19

European Working Group on Sarcopenia in Older People 2 (EWGSOP2)	*Asian Working Group for Sarcopenia (AWGS-2019)*
Sarcopenia is a progressive and generalized skeletal muscle disorder that is associated with increased likelihood of adverse outcomes including falls, fractures, physical disability, and mortality.	Age-related loss of skeletal muscle mass plus loss of muscle strength and/or reduced physical performance.

2010). Likewise, the Asian Working Group for Sarcopenia (AWGS) developed its own criteria, grounded in epidemiological data from East Asian populations, which also emphasize the combined evaluation of muscle mass, strength, and physical performance (Chen et al., 2014). These regional adaptations reflect an increasing acknowledgment of sarcopenia's effects on aging populations globally and the necessity for customized diagnostic criteria that consider specific demographic and ethnic characteristics.

In September 2016, the WHO included sarcopenia in the International Classification of Diseases 10 (ICD-10) (Anker et al., 2016), making it a widely accepted concept globally and recognizing it as a crucial biomarker for evaluating human health across various stages of the life cycle and in diverse clinical situations (Cruz-Jentoft & Sayer, 2019).

Both EWGSOP's and AWGS's definitions have undergone revisions, with the most recent updates in 2018 (EWGSOP2) (Cruz-Jentoft et al., 2019) and 2019 (AWGS-2019) (Chen et al., 2020). These updates emphasize the importance of muscle strength and physical performance as key criteria for diagnosing sarcopenia, underscoring their role in predicting adverse outcomes. Additionally, specific cut-off points for these parameters have been established. The definitions published by both groups are presented in Table 8.1.

In summary, sarcopenia has evolved from a concept focused solely on muscle loss to a complex syndrome characterized by diminished muscle mass, strength, and function. This shift has significant implications for the health and functioning of the elderly population. The broader perspective underscores the importance of comprehensive approaches, essential for developing targeted interventions like exercise and nutritional strategies. These interventions aim to manage and potentially reverse the effects of sarcopenia, thereby mitigating the adverse outcomes associated with this condition (Akishita et al., 2018).

Screening and Diagnosis

Like the concept of sarcopenia, the methods for its identification and diagnosis have evolved over time. Until 2010, the identification of sarcopenia primarily relied on the Appendicular Skeletal Muscle Index (ASMI) proposed by

Baumgartner and colleagues in 1998. This index measures body composition using an anthropometric equation that includes the sum of appendicular skeletal muscle mass (ASM) of both arms and legs in kilograms, and the individual's height in meters squared (ASMI = ASM kg/height^2 (m^2)). Sarcopenia was initially defined as an ASMI that is more than two standard deviations below the mean of a reference group of young adults (Baumgartner et al., 1998). However, according to the revised definition of sarcopenia by various international working groups, sarcopenia not only negatively affects an individual's muscle mass but also impacts muscle strength and, consequently, physical performance (Figure 8.1).

Approximately 40% of an individual's body weight corresponds to their muscle mass. From the age of 30, muscle mass decreases by 3% to 8% per

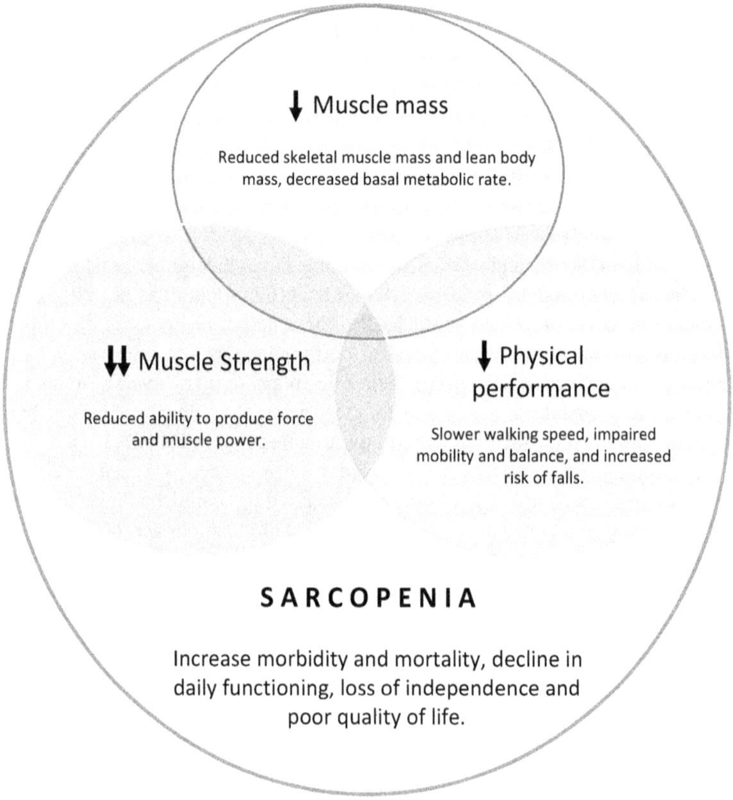

Figure 8.1 Impact of sarcopenia on muscle mass, strength, and physical performance according to revised definitions by international working groups.

decade of life, resulting in an average loss of approximately 0.2 kg of lean body mass per year (Forbes & Halloran, 1976). After the age of 50, the percentage of loss increases to 5%–10% per decade, or approximately 0.4 kg of lean body mass per year (Hughes et al., 2002). There is evidence that muscle mass plays an important role in reducing metabolic risk factors associated with cardiovascular diseases (Braith & Stewart, 2006; Hurley et al., 1988). In consequence, sarcopenia is associated with a decrease in physiological reserve, which can lead to pathological conditions such as osteoporosis (Nelson et al., 1994), decreased basal metabolic rate (Westcott, 2010), obesity (Strasser & Schobersberger, 2011), diabetes (Flack et al., 2010), metabolic syndrome (Strasser et al., 2010) and an increased risk of all-cause mortality (FitzGerald et al., 2004).

Muscle strength is defined as the maximum force generated by a muscle or muscle group at a specific speed. The ability to produce the force necessary for initiating and sustaining movement is a fundamental physiological and mechanical function of skeletal muscle. In older adults, there is a notable decline in muscle strength (Frontera et al., 2000). Muscle strength was shown to be a more potent predictor of clinically relevant outcomes than muscle mass alone, for three reasons. First, the age-related reduction in muscle strength occurs earlier than the reduction in muscle mass (Cruz-Jentoft & Sayer, 2019). Second, the rate of decline in muscle strength is greater than that of muscle mass (Cruz-Jentoft & Sayer, 2019). Lastly, the age-related loss of muscle strength cannot be solely explained by the reduction in muscle mass (Wilkinson et al., 2018).

Additionally, sarcopenia negatively impact the physical performance (Reid & Fielding, 2012) and mobility (Visser et al., 2005) of older adults. Physical performance has been established as an important predictor of adverse outcomes such as falls (Ward et al., 2015), difficulty or inability to perform daily living activities (Baumgartner et al., 1998), disability (Xie et al., 2020), depression, hospitalization (Guralnik et al., 2000), reduced independence (Tinetti & Williams, 1997) and quality of life (Beaudart et al., 2015), and even increased mortality in this population (Cruz-Jentoft et al., 2019).

In conclusion, nowadays, the screening and diagnosis of sarcopenia requires a comprehensive assessment that includes the evaluation of muscle strength, muscle mass, and physical performance. These three elements are critical indicators of sarcopenia and its impact on overall health. Therefore, assessments of body composition, such as ASMI, should always be accompanied by an evaluation of muscle strength when the aim is to detect or diagnose sarcopenia. Additionally, it is recommended to assess physical performance to determine the severity of sarcopenia (Chen et al., 2020; Cruz-Jentoft et al., 2010). A variety of tests and technologies are available to assess these elements, allowing for early detection and targeted interventions.

The EWGSOP2 and AWSG 2019 offers explicit guidelines on the cut-off points for each diagnostic measure, promoting a more uniform approach to diagnosing sarcopenia (Chen et al., 2020; Cruz-Jentoft et al., 2019). The cut-off

Table 8.2 Cut-off values proposed by EWDS2 and WAS 2018 for different diagnostic measures

Element	*Test*	*EWGSOP2*	*AWGS 2019*
Strength	Handgrip strength (kg)	M: <27; F: <16	**M: <28; F: <18**
Muscle Quantity	ASM (kg)	M: <20; F: <15	
	ASM/height^2 (kg/m^2)	M: <7.0; F: <5.5	**M: <7.0; F: <5.4**
Physical Performance	6-m walk speed (m/s)		**<1.0**
	Gait speed (m/s)	≤0.8	
	Five-time sit-to-stand (s)	>15	**≥12**
	Short physical performance battery (score)	≤8	**≤9**
	400 m walk (min)	Non-completion or ≥6	
	Time up and go (s)	≥20	

ASM: appendicular skeletal muscle mass; F: female; M: male.

points for these diagnostic tools differ depending on the population examined and the methodologies employed. Standardizing these cut-off points is crucial to maintaining consistency in sarcopenia diagnosis across various clinical and research settings. The cut-off points for the different diagnostic tests proposed by EWGSOP2 and AWGS 2019 are presented in Table 8.2.

Muscle Mass Measurement

Muscle quantity or mass can be evaluated using techniques like dual-energy X-ray absorptiometry (DXA), bioelectrical impedance analysis (BIA), or simple anthropometric measures such as body mass index (BMI) and calf circumference. Each method has its recommended cut-off points, which can vary widely depending on the population studied and the specific equipment used (Cruz-Jentoft et al., 2019).

Dual-energy X-ray Absorptiometry (DXA): this method is extensively used for evaluating muscle mass. DXA provides comprehensive measurements of muscle mass, fat mass, and bone mass, and is regarded as the gold standard for assessing total body composition (Tournadre et al., 2019). Specific cut-off points are used to identify low muscle mass, based on either total appendicular lean mass (ALM) (Cruz-Jentoft et al., 2019) or ALM divided by height squared (ALM/ht^2) (Chen et al., 2020; Cruz-Jentoft et al., 2019).

Bioelectrical Impedance Analysis (BIA): BIA is a cost-effective alternative to DXA for quickly measuring lean mass, though it does not directly assess the muscle and bone compartments. BIA values are influenced by the individual's hydration status, have not been validated in patients with chronic diseases, and tend to underestimate lean mass (Tournadre et al., 2019). Despite being less accurate than DXA, BIA offers a portable and more accessible option for estimating muscle mass in clinical settings.

Computed Tomography (CT) and Magnetic Resonance Imaging (MRI): These methods are regarded as gold standards in clinical research (Rossi et al., 2018). They provide high-quality images that enable precise differentiation between muscle and other tissues and are employed to measure muscle cross-sectional area (Goodpaster et al., 1997).

Muscle Strength

Muscle strength has been prioritized as the primary criterion for sarcopenia screening. Consequently, different assessments have been proposed to measure muscle strength in the geriatric population.

Isometric Dynamometry*:* Handgrip strength (HGS) is commonly employed as a primary indicator of isometric muscle strength in clinical practice due to its cost-effectiveness, simplicity, and portability. The EWGSOP2 and AWGS 2019 highlights the significance of HGS as a key marker for diagnosing sarcopenia, offering specific cut-off points (Table 8.2) (Chen et al., 2020; Cruz-Jentoft et al., 2019).

Physical Performance

Gait Speed Test: This test measures the time required to walk a specified distance. Slower walking speeds are correlated with an increased risk of adverse outcomes related to sarcopenia (Rossi et al., 2018). Gait speed is regarded as a dependable indicator of muscle function, with a common threshold of ≤ 0.8 m/s over six meters used to diagnose sarcopenia (Cruz-Jentoft et al., 2019; Nishikawa et al., 2021).

Short Physical Performance Battery (SPPB): This assessment evaluates lower extremity function through tasks such as balance tests, walking speed, and chair rise tests. The SPPB uses a scoring system where lower scores indicate poorer physical performance and greater severity of sarcopenia. It is widely used in clinical settings to assess physical performance (Rossi et al., 2018).

The Sit to Stand Test (STS): This test measures the time it takes a patient to stand up from a seated position five times without using their arms. As this test requires both strength and endurance, it serves as a proxy indicator of leg muscle strength, particularly the quadriceps muscle group. While AWGS 2019 considers the STS a physical performance test, the EWGSOP2 classifies it as a strength test (Chen et al., 2020; Cruz-Jentoft et al., 2019).

Timed Up and Go (TUG) Test: This assessment determines the time required for an individual to rise from a chair, walk a short distance, turn around, return to the chair, and sit down. It is utilized to evaluate mobility and balance (Rossi et al., 2018).

In summary, diagnosing sarcopenia requires a comprehensive approach that involves evaluating muscle strength, muscle mass, and physical performance. Employing standardized tools and cut-off points, as recommended by consensus groups such as EWGSOP2 and ASWG 2019, ensures accurate diagnosis and effective management of sarcopenia. The choice of tools and cut-off points depends on the clinical or research setting, equipment availability, and target population.

Combination of Measures in Diagnostic Algorithms

In recent years, specific criteria have been established for diagnosing sarcopenia. Both EWGSOP2 and AWGS 2019 suggest using algorithms that include a combination of the measures mentioned in the previous paragraphs in a sequential diagnostic process (Chen et al., 2020; Cruz-Jentoft et al., 2019). These algorithms can be very useful in the clinical setting to identify individuals with sarcopenia and to define the degree of severity of the condition. The diagnostic process generally begins with case finding, often using tools such as the SARC-F questionnaire or clinical observations indicating possible sarcopenia (e.g., functional decline, repeated falls, or chronic conditions). If the initial screening suggests risk, the next step involves assessing muscle strength using handgrip strength or the five-time chair stand test to confirm the diagnosis, and finally, an evaluation of physical performance to determine the degree of sarcopenia.

Case Finding

In clinical practice, sarcopenia screening may be initiated using tools such as the SARC-F questionnaire, or when a patient exhibits symptoms or signs indicative of the condition. The AWGS 2019 algorithm starts with recommendations for identifying cases if any of the following clinical conditions are present: (i) functional decline or limitations, unintentional weight loss, depressive mood, cognitive impairment, repeated falls, or malnutrition; or (ii) chronic conditions such as heart failure, chronic obstructive pulmonary disease, diabetes mellitus, and chronic kidney disease (Chen et al., 2020). The EWGSOP2 algorithm also begins the diagnostic process with case finding using the SARC-F questionnaire or clinical suspicion (Cruz-Jentoft et al., 2019). In these instances, it is advisable to conduct further tests to confirm the presence of sarcopenia. The specific criteria for case finding can be found in Table 8.3.

Table 8.3 Specific criteria for case finding

EWGS2		*AWGS 2019*	
Criteria	*Diagnosis*	*Criteria*	*Diagnosis*
SARC-F ≥ 4 OR clinical suspicion	Positive or present. Assess muscle strength	CC M: <34 cm; F: <33 cm **OR** SARC-F ≥ 4 **OR** SARC-Calf ≥ 11	Assess muscle strength or physical performance

CC: Calf circumference; M: male; F: female.

A widely recognized tool for detecting cases of sarcopenia is the SARC-F questionnaire, which includes five questions assessing strength, assistance with walking, rising from a chair, climbing stairs, and falls. Each question is scored from 0 to 2, yielding a total score ranging from 0 to 10 (Malmstrom & Morley, 2013). A score of ≥ 4 points indicates an increased risk of sarcopenia (Cruz-Jentoft et al., 2019; Nishikawa et al., 2021). The SARC-F is valued for its simplicity and high specificity, though it has been criticized for its low sensitivity, potentially missing many sarcopenia cases (Nishikawa et al., 2021). To enhance SARC-F's sensitivity, the SARC-CalF has been proposed, combining the SARC-F with calf circumference measurements. This approach has demonstrated improved screening performance and sensitivity compared to SARC-F alone. The optimal cut-off values for calf circumference are suggested to be <34 cm for men and <33 cm for women (Nishikawa et al., 2021).

Diagnosis

Once a high risk of sarcopenia is identified using the SARC-F questionnaire, the next steps should include evaluating muscle strength, measuring muscle mass, and finally, assessing physical performance. The selection of methods may vary based on the clinical or research context, the availability of equipment, and the specific requirements of the population under examination. If muscle strength is low, the diagnosis of "probable sarcopenia" is made, and further evaluation of muscle mass is required to confirm the condition. Methods such as DXA or BIA are typically employed to measure muscle mass. When both muscle strength and muscle mass are below the established cut-off points, the diagnosis is updated to "confirmed sarcopenia." Finally, physical performance is assessed to determine the severity of sarcopenia. Common tests include gait speed, the SPPB, or the TUG test. Severe limitations in physical performance, combined with low muscle mass and strength, indicate "severe sarcopenia."

This structured approach ensures that each diagnostic element contributes to a comprehensive understanding of the patient's condition, enabling tailored interventions. The specific diagnostic criteria, along with the recommended tools, assessment methods, and cut-off points, are detailed in Table 8.4.

New Insights on the Assessment of Strength for Health

Both the definition and assessment strategies for sarcopenia have evolved over the past two decades, and it is reasonable to anticipate further changes as ongoing research and technological advancements deepen our understanding of the condition. As the field progresses, there is a growing need for more precise evaluations to enhance the detection and diagnosis of sarcopenia, ensuring effective management and targeted interventions for affected individuals. HGS is proposed as the primary strength assessment for identifying sarcopenia, as multiple studies have determined that it serves as an indicative measure of

Table 8.4 Diagnostic criteria and resulting diagnoses from the application of sarcopenia algorithms

EWGS2			*AWGS 2019*		
Criteria	*Assessment*	*Diagnosis*	*Criteria*	*Assessment*	*Diagnosis*
Low muscle strength	Handgrip strength (M: <27 kg, F: <16 kg), five-time chair stand test (>15 s)	Probable sarcopenia	Low muscle strength **OR** low physical performance	Handgrip strength (M: <28 kg, F: <18 kg), 6 m walk (<1.0 m/s), five-time chair stand test (≥12 s), SPPB (≤9)	Possible sarcopenia
Low muscle strength *AND* low muscle mass	DXA, BIA, CT, MRI: ASM (M: <20 kg, F: <15 kg), ASM/height^2 M: <7.0 kg/m^2, F: <5.5 kg/m^2).	Confirmed sarcopenia	Low muscle mass **AND** low muscle strength **OR** low physical performance	DXA (M: <7.0 kg/m^2, F: <5.4 kg/m^2), BIA (M: <7.0 kg/m^2, F: <5.7 kg/m^2), Handgrip strength (M: <28 kg, F: <18 kg), 6 m walk (<1.0 m/s), five-time chair stand test (≥12 s), SPPB (≤9)	Sarcopenia
Low muscle strength, low muscle mass *AND* low physical performance	Gait speed (≤0.8 m/s), SPPB (≤8 point score), TUG (≥20 s), 400 m walk (non-completion or ≥6 min for completion)	Severe sarcopenia	Low muscle mass **AND** low muscle strength **AND** low physical performance	DXA, BIA, Handgrip strength, 6 m walk, five-time chair stand test, SPPB	Severe sarcopenia

BIA: Bioelectrical Impedance Analysis; CT: Computed Tomography; DXA: Dual-Energy X-Ray Absorptiometry; SPPB: Short Physical Performance Battery; TUG: Timed Up and Go; M: male; F: female.

overall muscle strength, physical performance and is predictive of key clinical outcomes (Rossi et al., 2018). However, several aspects remain unresolved, and there is controversy regarding the use of HGS for assessing overall muscle strength. For instance, there are contrasting findings regarding the association between HGS and isometric knee extension and flexion strength (Tatangelo et al., 2022). Handgrip strength measurement primarily assesses the muscles of the upper limbs and may not fully reflect the strength status of the lower limbs. Additionally, the decline in muscle function appears to be less pronounced in the upper limb muscles compared to the muscle groups of the lower limbs (Rodacki et al., 2020). Similarly, data on the association between HGS and physical performance are contradictory (Tatangelo et al., 2022). The EWGSOP2 recommends using isometric torque methods to measure lower limb strength when assessing grip strength is not feasible due to hand impairment. However, it does not establish specific cut-off points for lower limb strength. Given the crucial role of lower limb strength, particularly that of the extensor muscles, in various functional tasks, the measurement of knee extension strength is a key issue. For this purpose, angular isokinetic dynamometry has long been considered the gold standard method for assessing dynamic muscle strength (Dvir & Müller, 2020). This technique assesses muscle strength using devices that regulate the speed of muscle contraction while simultaneously measuring the force exerted, and its use is feasible in frail older adults (Callahan et al., 2007). According to the systematic review by Steffl and Stastny (2020), the isokinetic knee extension strength values at 60°/s that can identify sarcopenia are 83 ± 23 Nm in men and 60 ± 7 Nm in women. For knee flexion, the corresponding values are 47 ± 6 Nm for men and 36 ± 5 Nm for women (Steffl & Stastny, 2020). While this methodology delivers highly accurate strength measurements, its relevance to daily activities is limited as it only assesses isolated, single-joint movements (Piche et al., 2021). To accurately predict physical performance and assess the risk of falls, it is essential to evaluate lower limb strength rather than focusing solely on isolated muscle groups (Rodacki et al., 2020). Alternative methods, such as the leg press using the Nottingham leg power rig, have been employed to evaluate lower limb muscle strength in multi-joint actions (Alcazar et al., 2017; Lindemann et al., 2003). However, the guidance provided by these devices during movement removes the need for coordination and balance, which are essential for everyday activities. In this context, Alcazar et al. (2018) devised a formula validated for assessing mean mechanical power in the lower limbs of older adults, based on their performance in the five-time chair stand test (Alcazar et al., 2018). Five-time chair stand test involves lower limb movement, joint coordination, postural control, and the generation of isometric, dynamic, and power strength (Lindemann et al., 2007). This movement has demonstrated strong associations with measures of physical function (Baltasar-Fernandez et al., 2021), balance (Bohannon, 2012), and fall risk (Cho et al., 2012) in older adults. Alcazar et al.'s formula utilizes anthropometric measurements, biomechanical principles, and the time taken to complete five-time chair stand test to estimate mean mechanical power. Validation of this method was conducted using a force platform (Baltasar-Fernandez et al., 2021). One of the noteworthy aspects of Alcazar et al.'s method is that it measures lower limb power, which has been established as one of the primary predictors of physical performance in older adults (Reid & Fielding, 2012).

Muscle Power: A Key Determinant of Physical Performance in Older Adults

Early research focused on muscle strength in older adults (Aniansson et al., 1980), but recent studies underscore the significance of muscle power (Reid & Fielding, 2012). Muscle power declines earlier and at a faster rate than muscle strength (Kennis et al., 2014), impacting balance and mobility (Bassey et al., 1992; Bean et al., 2003), and increasing fall risk (Perry et al., 2007). While strength denotes the maximum force muscles can exert, power is defined as the force generated quickly (power = force × velocity) (Caserotti, 2010). Moreover, some researchers argue that contraction speed better predicts performance in tasks such as walking (Sayers et al., 2005), rising from a chair, climbing stairs (Cuoco et al., 2004), and maintaining balance (Mayson et al., 2008). Therefore, muscle power is now recognized as a critical determinant of functional capacity in older adults (Reid & Fielding, 2012). Due to the necessity to objectively measure force, velocity, and power variables during multi-joint functional gestures, the utilization of functional electromechanical dynamometry (FEMD) is gradually increasing, and its reliability and validity have been evaluated (Del-Cuerpo et al., 2023; Jerez-Mayorga et al., 2021; Reyes-Ferrada et al., 2022; Rodriguez-Perea et al., 2021). Jerez-Mayorga et al. (2021) evaluated the reliability of the strength and velocity of movement of the concentric phase of the five-time chair stand test measured by a FEMD during different conditions (5 kg, 10 kg and 15 kg) in healthy young adults (Jerez-Mayorga et al., 2021). They reported CV values of 2.84, 1.80, and 3.11 for Average Velocity at 5 kg, 10 kg, and 15 kg conditions, respectively. The findings suggest that the FEMD can provide consistent and reliable assessments of movement velocity during the five-time chair stand test across varying loads. Such assessments would be highly valuable in geriatrics for accurately evaluating the physical performance of older adults. *Role of Rate of Force Development (RFD) in Fall Prevention and Frailty Assessment Among Older Adults*. The rate of force development (RFD), which measures the force generated within the initial 200 ms of muscle contraction (Aagaard et al., 2002), is critical for fall prevention (Maki & McIlroy, 2006). Deficits in RFD observed in older adults, coupled with the nature of falls, may explain the role of muscle power in preventing them. Older adults exhibit RFD deficits significantly higher than those in maximal strength, with RFD being 51.2% lower than in young subjects (Häkkinen & Häkkinen, 1991). A recent study estimated that falls from standing occur within 0.27 to 0.63 seconds, which is a rapid and dynamic process

(Qiao & Yang, 2020). Corrective actions such as recovery steps and applying necessary force must be executed swiftly (Maki & McIlroy, 2006), highlighting reactive balance as the ultimate defense against falls (Kim et al., 2021). Given that increased falls are a consequence of sarcopenia, which ranks as the second leading cause of injury-related death among older adults, RFD should be considered a critical variable in assessing frailty in this population. In conclusion, current methodologies for assessing strength, primarily HGS, have limitations in evaluating overall muscle strength and correlating it with lower limb strength and physical performance. Recognizing the critical role of lower limb strength and power, especially in multi-joint functional tasks, underscores the importance of adopting new methodologies that integrate the assessment of strength, velocity, and power variables during functional gestures. These advancements will enhance our understanding of sarcopenia risk and related conditions in older populations.

References

Aagaard, P., Simonsen, E. B., Andersen, J. L., Magnusson, P., & Dyhre-Poulsen, P. (2002). Increased rate of force development and neural drive of human skeletal muscle following resistance training. *Journal of Applied Physiology (Bethesda, Md. : 1985)*, 93(4), 1318–1326. https://doi.org/10.1152/japplphysiol.00283.2002

Akishita, M., Kozaki, K., Iijima, K., Tanaka, T., Shibasaki, K., Ogawa, S., & Arai, H. (2018). Chapter 1 Definitions and diagnosis of sarcopenia. *Geriatrics & Gerontology International*, 18(Suppl 1), 7–12. https://doi.org/10.1111/ggi.13311

Alcazar, J., Losa-Reyna, J., Rodriguez-Lopez, C., Alfaro-Acha, A., Rodriguez-Mañas, L., Ara, I., García-García, F. J., & Alegre, L. M. (2018). The sit-to-stand muscle power test: An easy, inexpensive and portable procedure to assess muscle power in older people. *Experimental Gerontology*, 112, 38–43. https://doi.org/10.1016/j.exger.2018.08.006

Alcazar, J., Rodriguez-Lopez, C., Ara, I., Alfaro-Acha, A., Mañas-Bote, A., Guadalupe-Grau, A., García-García, F. J., & Alegre, L. M. (2017). The force-velocity relationship in older people: Reliability and validity of a systematic procedure. *International Journal of Sports Medicine*, 38(14), 1097–1104. https://doi.org/10.1055/s-0043-119880

Aniansson, A., Rundgren, A., & Sperling, L. (1980). Evaluation of functional capacity in activities of daily living in 70-year-old men and women. *Scandinavian Journal of Rehabilitation Medicine*, 12(4), 145–154.

Anker, S. D., Morley, J. E., & von Haehling, S. (2016). Welcome to the ICD-10 code for sarcopenia. *Journal of Cachexia, Sarcopenia and Muscle*, 7(5), 512–514. https://doi.org/10.1002/jcsm.12147

Baltasar-Fernandez, I., Alcazar, J., Rodriguez-Lopez, C., Losa-Reyna, J., Alonso-Seco, M., Ara, I., & Alegre, L. M. (2021). Sit-to-stand muscle power test: Comparison between estimated and force plate-derived mechanical power and their association with physical function in older adults. *Experimental Gerontology*, 145, 111213. https://doi.org/10.1016/j.exger.2020.111213

Bassey, E. J., Fiatarone, M. A., O'Neill, E. F., Kelly, M., Evans, W. J., & Lipsitz, L. A. (1992). Leg extensor power and functional performance in very old men and women. *Clinical Science (London, England : 1979)*, 82(3), 321–327. https://doi.org/10.1042/cs0820321

Bauer, J., Morley, J. E., Schols, A. M. W. J., Ferrucci, L., Cruz-Jentoft, A. J., Dent, E., Baracos, V. E., Crawford, J. A., Doehner, W., Heymsfield, S. B., Jatoi, A., Kalantar-Zadeh, K., Lainscak, M., Landi, F., Laviano, A., Mancuso, M., Muscaritoli, M., Prado, C. M., Strasser, F., . . . Anker, S. D. (2019). Sarcopenia: A time for action. An SCWD position paper. *Journal of Cachexia, Sarcopenia and Muscle*, 10(5), 956–961. https://doi.org/10.1002/jcsm.12483

Baumgartner, R. N., Koehler, K. M., Gallagher, D., Romero, L., Heymsfield, S. B., Ross, R. R., Garry, P. J., & Lindeman, R. D. (1998). Epidemiology of sarcopenia among the elderly in New Mexico. *American Journal of Epidemiology*, 147(8), 755–763. https://doi.org/10.1093/oxfordjournals.aje.a009520

Bean, J. F., Leveille, S. G., Kiely, D. K., Bandinelli, S., Guralnik, J. M., & Ferrucci, L. (2003). A comparison of leg power and leg strength within the InCHIANTI study: Which influences mobility more? *The Journals of Gerontology. Series A, Biological Sciences and Medical Sciences*, 58(8), 728–733. https://doi.org/10.1093/gerona/58.8.m728

Beaudart, C., Reginster, J. Y., Petermans, J., Gillain, S., Quabron, A., Locquet, M., Slomian, J., Buckinx, F., & Bruyère, O. (2015). Quality of life and physical components linked to sarcopenia: The SarcoPhAge study. *Experimental Gerontology*, 69, 103–110. https://doi.org/10.1016/j.exger.2015.05.003

Bohannon, R. W. (2012). Measurement of sit-to-stand among older adults. *Topics in Geriatric Rehabilitation*, 28(1), 11–16.

Braith, R. W., & Stewart, K. J. (2006). Resistance exercise training: Its role in the prevention of cardiovascular disease. *Circulation*, 113(22), 2642–2450. https://doi.org/10.1161/CIRCULATIONAHA.105.584060/ASSET/827698C0-2819-44D5-8D5F-BC50DA478666/ASSETS/GRAPHIC/13FF1.JPEG

Briggs, A. M., Cross, M. J., Hoy, D. G., Sànchez-Riera, L., Blyth, F. M., Woolf, A. D., & March, L. (2016). Musculoskeletal health conditions represent a global threat to healthy aging: A Report for the 2015 World Health Organization world report on ageing and health. *The Gerontologist*, 56(Suppl 2), S243–55. https://doi.org/10.1093/geront/gnw002

Callahan, D., Phillips, E., Carabello, R., Frontera, W. R., & Fielding, R. A. (2007). Assessment of lower extremity muscle power in functionally-limited elders. *Aging Clinical and Experimental Research*, 19(3), 194–199. https://doi.org/10.1007/BF03324689

Caserotti, P. (2010). Strength training in older adults: Changes in mechanical muscle function and functional performance. *Open Sports Sciences Journal*, 3(1), 62–66.

Chang, K.-V., Hsu, T.-H., Wu, W.-T., Huang, K.-C., & Han, D.-S. (2017). Is sarcopenia associated with depression? A systematic review and meta-analysis of observational studies. *Age and Ageing*, 46(5), 738–746.

Chen, L.-K., Liu, L.-K., Woo, J., Assantachai, P., Auyeung, T.-W., Bahyah, K. S., Chou, M.-Y., Chen, L.-Y., Hsu, P.-S., Krairit, O., Lee, J. S. W., Lee, W.-J., Lee, Y., Liang, C.-K., Limpawattana, P., Lin, C.-S., Peng, L.-N.,

Satake, S., Suzuki, T., . . . Arai, H. (2014). Sarcopenia in Asia: Consensus report of the Asian Working Group for Sarcopenia. *Journal of the American Medical Directors Association*, 15(2), 95–101. https://doi.org/10.1016/j.jamda.2013.11.025

Chen, L.-K., Woo, J., Assantachai, P., Auyeung, T.-W., Chou, M.-Y., Iijima, K., Jang, H. C., Kang, L., Kim, M., Kim, S., Kojima, T., Kuzuya, M., Lee, J. S. W., Lee, S. Y., Lee, W.-J., Lee, Y., Liang, C.-K., Lim, J.-Y., Lim, W. S., . . . Arai, H. (2020). Asian Working Group for Sarcopenia: 2019 consensus update on sarcopenia diagnosis and treatment. *Journal of the American Medical Directors Association*, 21(3), 300–307.e2. https://doi.org/10.1016/j.jamda.2019.12.012

Cho, K. H., Bok, S. K., Kim, Y.-J., & Hwang, S. L. (2012). Effect of lower limb strength on falls and balance of the elderly. *Annals of Rehabilitation Medicine*, 36(3), 386–393. https://doi.org/10.5535/arm.2012.36.3.386

Clark, B. C., & Manini, T. M. (2008). Sarcopenia =/= dynapenia. *The Journals of Gerontology. Series A, Biological Sciences and Medical Sciences*, 63(8), 829–834. https://doi.org/10.1093/gerona/63.8.829

Cruz-Jentoft, A. J., Baeyens, J. P., Bauer, J. M., Boirie, Y., Cederholm, T., Landi, F., Martin, F. C., Michel, J.-P., Rolland, Y., Schneider, S. M., Topinková, E., Vandewoude, M., & Zamboni, M. (2010). Sarcopenia: European consensus on definition and diagnosis: Report of the European Working Group on Sarcopenia in Older People. *Age and Ageing*, 39(4), 412–423. https://doi.org/10.1093/ageing/afq034

Cruz-Jentoft, A. J., Bahat, G., Bauer, J., Boirie, Y., Bruyère, O., Cederholm, T., Cooper, C., Landi, F., Rolland, Y., Sayer, A. A., Schneider, S. M., Sieber, C. C., Topinkova, E., Vandewoude, M., Visser, M., & Zamboni, M. (2019). Sarcopenia: Revised European consensus on definition and diagnosis. *Age and Ageing*, 48(1), 16–31. https://doi.org/10.1093/ageing/afy169

Cruz-Jentoft, A. J., & Sayer, A. A. (2019). Sarcopenia. *Lancet (London, England)*, 393(10191), 2636–2646. https://doi.org/10.1016/S0140-6736(19)31138-9

Cuoco, A., Callahan, D. M., Sayers, S., Frontera, W. R., Bean, J., & Fielding, R. A. (2004). Impact of muscle power and force on gait speed in disabled older men and women. *The Journals of Gerontology. Series A, Biological Sciences and Medical Sciences*, 59(11), 1200–1206. https://doi.org/10.1093/gerona/59.11.1200

Del-Cuerpo, I., Jerez-Mayorga, D., Delgado-Floody, P., Morenas-Aguilar, M. D., & Chirosa-Ríos, L. J. (2023). Test-retest reliability of the functional electromechanical dynamometer for squat exercise. *International Journal of Environmental Research and Public Health*, 20(2). https://doi.org/10.3390/ijerph20021289

Dvir, Z., & Müller, S. (2020). Multiple-joint isokinetic dynamometry: A critical review. *Journal of Strength and Conditioning Research*, 34(2), 587–601. https://doi.org/10.1519/JSC.0000000000002982

Evans, W. J. (1995). What is sarcopenia? *The Journals of Gerontology. Series A, Biological Sciences and Medical Sciences*, 50 Spec No, 5–8. https://doi.org/10.1093/gerona/50a.special_issue.5

Fielding, R. A., Vellas, B., Evans, W. J., Bhasin, S., Morley, J. E., Newman, A. B., Abellan van Kan, G., Andrieu, S., Bauer, J., Breuille, D., Cederholm, T.,

Chandler, J., De Meynard, C., Donini, L., Harris, T., Kannt, A., Keime Guibert, F., Onder, G., Papanicolaou, D., . . . Zamboni, M. (2011). Sarcopenia: An undiagnosed condition in older adults. Current consensus definition: Prevalence, etiology, and consequences. International working group on sarcopenia. *Journal of the American Medical Directors Association*, 12(4), 249–256. https://doi.org/10.1016/j.jamda.2011.01.003

FitzGerald, S. J., Barlow, C. E., Kampert, J. B., Morrow, J. R., Jackson, A. W., & Blair, S. N. (2004). Muscular fitness and all-cause mortality: Prospective observations. *Journal of Physical Activity and Health*, 1(1), 7–18.

Flack, K. D., Davy, K. P., Hulver, M. W., Winett, R. A., Frisard, M. I., & Davy, B. M. (2010). Aging, resistance training, and diabetes prevention. *Journal of Aging Research*, 2011, 127315. https://doi.org/10.4061/2011/127315

Forbes, G. B., & Halloran, E. (1976). The adult decline in lean body mass. *Human Biology*, 48(1), 161–173.

Fried, L. P., Tangen, C. M., Walston, J., Newman, A. B., Hirsch, C., Gottdiener, J., Seeman, T., Tracy, R., Kop, W. J., Burke, G., & McBurnie, M. A. (2001). Frailty in older adults: Evidence for a phenotype. *The Journals of Gerontology. Series A, Biological Sciences and Medical Sciences*, 56(3), M146–56. https://doi.org/10.1093/gerona/56.3.m146

Frontera, W. R. (2022). Rehabilitation of older adults with sarcopenia: From cell to functioning. *Progress in Rehabilitation Medicine*, 7, 20220044. https://doi.org/10.2490/prm.20220044

Frontera, W. R., Hughes, V. A., Fielding, R. A., Fiatarone, M. A., Evans, W. J., & Roubenoff, R. (2000). Aging of skeletal muscle: A 12-yr longitudinal study. *Journal of Applied Physiology*, 88(4), 1321–1326.

Goodpaster, B. H., Thaete, F. L., Simoneau, J. A., & Kelley, D. E. (1997). Subcutaneous abdominal fat and thigh muscle composition predict insulin sensitivity independently of visceral fat. *Diabetes*, 46(10), 1579–1585. https://doi.org/10.2337/diacare.46.10.1579

Guralnik, J. M., Ferrucci, L., Pieper, C. F., Leveille, S. G., Markides, K. S., Ostir, G. V, Studenski, S., Berkman, L. F., & Wallace, R. B. (2000). Lower extremity function and subsequent disability: Consistency across studies, predictive models, and value of gait speed alone compared with the short physical performance battery. *The Journals of Gerontology. Series A, Biological Sciences and Medical Sciences*, 55(4), M221–31. https://doi.org/10.1093/gerona/55.4.m221

Häkkinen, K., & Häkkinen, A. (1991). Muscle cross-sectional area, force production and relaxation characteristics in women at different ages. *European Journal of Applied Physiology and Occupational Physiology*, 62(6), 410–414. https://doi.org/10.1007/BF00626612

Hong, S., Chang, Y., Jung, H.-S., Yun, K. E., Shin, H., & Ryu, S. (2017). Relative muscle mass and the risk of incident type 2 diabetes: A cohort study. *PloS One*, 12(11), e0188650.

Hughes, V. A., Frontera, W. R., Roubenoff, R., Evans, W. J., & Singh, M. A. F. (2002). Longitudinal changes in body composition in older men and women: Role of body weight change and physical activity. *The American Journal of Clinical Nutrition*, 76(2), 473–481. https://doi.org/10.1093/ajcn/76.2.473

Hurley, B. F., Hagberg, J. M., Goldberg, A. P., Seals, D. R., Ehsani, A. A., Brennan, R. E., & Holloszy, J. O. (1988). Resistive training can reduce coronary risk factors without altering VO2max or percent body fat. *Medicine and Science in Sports and Exercise*, 20(2), 150–154. https://doi.org/10.1249/00005768-198820020-00008

Jakovljevic, D. G. (2018). Physical activity and cardiovascular aging: Physiological and molecular insights. *Experimental Gerontology*, 109, 67–74.

Jerez-Mayorga, D., Huerta-Ojeda, Á., Chirosa-Ríos, L. J., Guede-Rojas, F., Guzmán-Guzmán, I. P., Intelangelo, L., Miranda-Fuentes, C., & Delgado-Floody, P. (2021). Test-retest reliability of functional electromechanical dynamometer on five sit-to-stand measures in healthy young adults. *International Journal of Environmental Research and Public Health*, 18(13). https://doi.org/10.3390/ijerph18136829

Jun, J. E., Choi, M. S., Park, S. W., Kim, G., Jin, S.-M., Kim, K., Hwang, Y.-C., Ahn, K. J., Chung, H. Y., & Jeong, I.-K. (2021). Low skeletal muscle mass is associated with the presence, incidence, and progression of coronary artery calcification. *Canadian Journal of Cardiology*, 37(9), 1480–1488.

Kennis, E., Verschueren, S., Van Roie, E., Thomis, M., Lefevre, J., & Delecluse, C. (2014). Longitudinal impact of aging on muscle quality in middle-aged men. *Age (Dordrecht, Netherlands)*, 36(4), 9689. https://doi.org/10.1007/s11357-014-9689-1

Kim, Y., Vakula, M. N., Bolton, D. A. E., Dakin, C. J., Thompson, B. J., Slocum, T. A., Teramoto, M., & Bressel, E. (2021). Which exercise interventions can most effectively improve reactive balance in older adults? A systematic review and network meta-analysis. In *Frontiers in aging neuroscience* (Vol. 13, p. 764826). https://doi.org/10.3389/fnagi.2021.764826

Lindemann, U., Claus, H., Stuber, M., Augat, P., Muche, R., Nikolaus, T., & Becker, C. (2003). Measuring power during the sit-to-stand transfer. *European Journal of Applied Physiology*, 89(5), 466–470. https://doi.org/10.1007/s00421-003-0837-z

Lindemann, U., Muche, R., Stuber, M., Zijlstra, W., Hauer, K., & Becker, C. (2007). Coordination of strength exertion during the chair-rise movement in very old people. *The Journals of Gerontology. Series A, Biological Sciences and Medical Sciences*, 62(6), 636–640. https://doi.org/10.1093/gerona/62.6.636

Maki, B. E., & McIlroy, W. E. (2006). Control of rapid limb movements for balance recovery: Age-related changes and implications for fall prevention. *Age and Ageing*, 35(Suppl 2), ii12–ii18. https://doi.org/10.1093/ageing/afl078

Malmstrom, T. K., & Morley, J. E. (2013). SARC-F: A simple questionnaire to rapidly diagnose sarcopenia. *Journal of the American Medical Directors Association*, 14(8), 531–532.

Marcell, T. J. (2003). Sarcopenia: Causes, consequences, and preventions. *The Journals of Gerontology. Series A, Biological Sciences and Medical Sciences*, 58(10), M911–6. https://doi.org/10.1093/gerona/58.10.m911

Martien, S., Delecluse, C., Boen, F., Seghers, J., Pelssers, J., Van Hoecke, A.-S., & Van Roie, E. (2015). Is knee extension strength a better predictor of functional performance than handgrip strength among older adults in three different settings? *Archives of Gerontology and Geriatrics*, 60(2), 252–258. https://doi.org/10.1016/j.archger.2014.11.010

Mayson, D. J., Kiely, D. K., LaRose, S. I., & Bean, J. F. (2008). Leg strength or velocity of movement: Which is more influential on the balance of mobility limited elders? *American Journal of Physical Medicine & Rehabilitation*, 87(12), 969–976. https://doi.org/10.1097/PHM.0b013e31818dfee5

Mijnarends, D. M., Luiking, Y. C., Halfens, R. J. G., Evers, S. M. A. A., Lenaerts, E. L. A., Verlaan, S., Wallace, M., Schols, J. M. G. A., & Meijers, J. M. M. (2018). Muscle, health and costs: A glance at their relationship. *The Journal of Nutrition, Health & Aging*, 22(7), 766–773. https://doi.org/10.1007/s12603-018-1058-9

Morley, J. E., Abbatecola, A. M., Argiles, J. M., Baracos, V., Bauer, J., Bhasin, S., Cederholm, T., Coats, A. J. S., Cummings, S. R., Evans, W. J., Fearon, K., Ferrucci, L., Fielding, R. A., Guralnik, J. M., Harris, T. B., Inui, A., Kalantar-Zadeh, K., Kirwan, B.-A., Mantovani, G., . . . Anker, S. D. (2011). Sarcopenia with limited mobility: An international consensus. *Journal of the American Medical Directors Association*, 12(6), 403–409. https://doi.org/10.1016/j.jamda.2011.04.014

Muscaritoli, M., Anker, S. D., Argilés, J., Aversa, Z., Bauer, J. M., Biolo, G., Boirie, Y., Bosaeus, I., Cederholm, T., Costelli, P., Fearon, K. C., Laviano, A., Maggio, M., Rossi Fanelli, F., Schneider, S. M., Schols, A., & Sieber, C. C. (2010). Consensus definition of sarcopenia, cachexia and pre-cachexia: Joint document elaborated by Special Interest Groups (SIG) "cachexia-anorexia in chronic wasting diseases" and "nutrition in geriatrics". *Clinical Nutrition (Edinburgh, Scotland)*, 29(2), 154–159. https://doi.org/10.1016/j.clnu.2009.12.004

Nelson, M. E., Fiatarone, M. A., Morganti, C. M., Trice, I., Greenberg, R. A., & Evans, W. J. (1994). Effects of high-intensity strength training on multiple risk factors for osteoporotic fractures. A randomized controlled trial. *JAMA*, 272(24), 1909–1914. https://doi.org/10.1001/jama.1994.03520240037038

Nishikawa, H., Asai, A., Fukunishi, S., Takeuchi, T., Goto, M., Ogura, T., Nakamura, S., Kakimoto, K., Miyazaki, T., Nishiguchi, S., & Higuchi, K. (2021). Screening Tools for Sarcopenia. *In Vivo (Athens, Greece)*, 35(6), 3001–3009. https://doi.org/10.21873/invivo.12595

O'Caoimh, R., Sezgin, D., O'Donovan, M. R., Molloy, D. W., Clegg, A., Rockwood, K., & Liew, A. (2021). Prevalence of frailty in 62 countries across the world: A systematic review and meta-analysis of population-level studies. *Age and Ageing*, 50(1), 96–104. https://doi.org/10.1093/ageing/afaa219

Perry, M. C., Carville, S. F., Smith, I. C. H., Rutherford, O. M., & Newham, D. J. (2007). Strength, power output and symmetry of leg muscles: Effect of age and history of falling. *European Journal of Applied Physiology*, 100(5), 553–561. https://doi.org/10.1007/s00421-006-0247-0

Piche, E., Chorin, F., Gerus, P., Jaafar, A., Reneaud, N., Guerin, O., & Zory, R. (2021). Validity of a simple sit-to-stand method for assessing force-velocity profile in older adults. *Experimental Gerontology*, 156, 111595. https://doi.org/10.1016/j.exger.2021.111595

Qiao, M., & Yang, F. (2020). Leg joint stiffness affects dynamics of backward falling from standing height: A simulation work. *Journal of Biomechanical Engineering*, 142(10). https://doi.org/10.1115/1.4047077

Reid, K. F., & Fielding, R. A. (2012). Skeletal muscle power: A critical determinant of physical functioning in older adults. *Exercise and Sport Sciences Reviews*, 40(1), 4–12.

Reyes-Ferrada, W., Chirosa-Ríos, L., Chirosa-Ríos, I., Martínez-García, D., Barboza-Gonzalez, P., Ulloa-Díaz, D., Jerez-Mayorga, D., & Rodríguez-Perea, Á. (2022). A new reliable device to assess trunk extensors strength. *Acta of Bioengineering and Biomechanics*, 24(1), 49–57.

Rodacki, A. L. F., Boneti Moreira, N., Pitta, A., Wolf, R., Melo Filho, J., Rodacki, C. de L. N., & Pereira, G. (2020). Is handgrip strength a useful measure to evaluate lower limb strength and functional performance in older women? *Clinical Interventions in Aging*, 15, 1045–1056. https://doi.org/10.2147/CIA.S253262

Rodriguez-Perea, A., Jerez-Mayorga, D., García-Ramos, A., Martínez-García, D., & Chirosa Rios, L. J. (2021). Reliability and concurrent validity of a functional electromechanical dynamometer device for the assessment of movement velocity. *Proceedings of the Institution of Mechanical Engineers, Part P: Journal of Sports Engineering and Technology*, 235(3), 176–181.

Rosenberg, I. H. (1997). Sarcopenia: Origins and clinical relevance. *The Journal of Nutrition*, 127(5 Suppl), 990S-991S. https://doi.org/10.1093/jn/127.5.990S

Rossi, A. P., Rubele, S., D'Introno, A., Zoico, E., Brandimarte, P., Amadio, G., Nori, N., Gnerre, P., Mazzali, G., & Fantin, F. (2018). An update on methods for sarcopenia diagnosis: From bench to bedside. *Italian Journal of Medicine*, 12(2), 97–107.

Roubenoff, R., & Hughes, V. A. (2000). Sarcopenia: Current concepts. *The Journals of Gerontology. Series A, Biological Sciences and Medical Sciences*, 55(12), M716–24. https://doi.org/10.1093/gerona/55.12.m716

Sayer, A. A., Syddall, H., Martin, H., Patel, H., Baylis, D., & Cooper, C. (2008). The developmental origins of sarcopenia. *The Journal of Nutrition, Health & Aging*, 12(7), 427–432. https://doi.org/10.1007/BF02982703

Sayers, S. P., Guralnik, J. M., Thombs, L. A., & Fielding, R. A. (2005). Effect of leg muscle contraction velocity on functional performance in older men and women. *Journal of the American Geriatrics Society*, 53(3), 467–471. https://doi.org/10.1111/j.1532-5415.2005.53166.x

Steffl, M., & Stastny, P. (2020). Isokinetic testing of muscle strength of older individuals with sarcopenia or frailty: A systematic review. *Isokinetics and Exercise Science*, 28(3), 291–301. https://doi.org/10.3233/IES-201148

Strasser, B., & Schobersberger, W. (2011). Evidence for resistance training as a treatment therapy in obesity. *Journal of Obesity*, 2011. https://doi.org/10.1155/2011/482564

Strasser, B., Siebert, U., & Schobersberger, W. (2010). Resistance training in the treatment of the metabolic syndrome: A systematic review and meta-analysis of the effect of resistance training on metabolic clustering in patients with abnormal glucose metabolism. *Sports Medicine (Auckland, N.Z.)*, 40(5), 397–415. https://doi.org/10.2165/11531380-000000000-00000

Studenski, S. A., Peters, K. W., Alley, D. E., Cawthon, P. M., McLean, R. R., Harris, T. B., Ferrucci, L., Guralnik, J. M., Fragala, M. S., Kenny, A. M., Kiel, D. P., Kritchevsky, S. B., Shardell, M. D., Dam, T.-T. L., & Vassileva,

M. T. (2014). The FNIH sarcopenia project: Rationale, study description, conference recommendations, and final estimates. *The Journals of Gerontology. Series A, Biological Sciences and Medical Sciences*, 69(5), 547–558. https://doi.org/10.1093/gerona/glu010

Tatangelo, T., Muollo, V., Ghiotto, L., Schena, F., & Rossi, A. P. (2022). Exploring the association between handgrip, lower limb muscle strength, and physical function in older adults: A narrative review. *Experimental Gerontology*, 167, 111902. https://doi.org/10.1016/j.exger.2022.111902

Tinetti, M. E., & Williams, C. S. (1997). Falls, injuries due to falls, and the risk of admission to a nursing home. *The New England Journal of Medicine*, 337(18), 1279–1284. https://doi.org/10.1056/NEJM199710303371806

Tournadre, A., Vial, G., Capel, F., Soubrier, M., & Boirie, Y. (2019). Sarcopenia. *Joint Bone Spine*, 86(3), 309–314.

United Nations. (2019*). United Nations World Population Prospects 2019 revision*. https://population.un.org/wpp/

Visser, M., Goodpaster, B. H., Kritchevsky, S. B., Newman, A. B., Nevitt, M., Rubin, S. M., Simonsick, E. M., & Harris, T. B. (2005). Muscle mass, muscle strength, and muscle fat infiltration as predictors of incident mobility limitations in well-functioning older persons. *The Journals of Gerontology. Series A, Biological Sciences and Medical Sciences*, 60(3), 324–333. https://doi.org/10.1093/gerona/60.3.324

Ward, R. E., Leveille, S. G., Beauchamp, M. K., Travison, T., Alexander, N., Jette, A. M., & Bean, J. F. (2015). Functional performance as a predictor of injurious falls in older adults. *Journal of the American Geriatrics Society*, 63(2), 315–320. https://doi.org/10.1111/jgs.13203

Westcott, W. L. (2010). Effects of strength training on resting energy expenditure. *American College of Sports Medicine Certified News*, 20, 10–11.

Wilkinson, D. J., Piasecki, M., & Atherton, P. J. (2018). The age-related loss of skeletal muscle mass and function: Measurement and physiology of muscle fibre atrophy and muscle fibre loss in humans. *Ageing Research Reviews*, 47, 123–132. https://doi.org/10.1016/j.arr.2018.07.005

World Health Organization. (2014). *Global status report on noncommunicable diseases 2014*. WHO Press. www.who.int/publications/i/item/9789241564854

World Health Organization. (2015). *World report on ageing and health*. World Health Organization.

Xie, W.-Q., Xiao, G.-L., Hu, P.-W., He, Y.-Q., Lv, S., & Xiao, W.-F. (2020). Possible sarcopenia: Early screening and intervention-narrative review. *Annals of Palliative Medicine*, 9(6), 4283–4293. https://doi.org/10.21037/apm-20-967

9 Evaluation of Muscle Quality

Daniel Jerez-Mayorga and Daniel Jiménez-Lupión

Conceptualization of Muscle Quality

Muscle quality, a comprehensive concept in exercise science, reflects not only the quantity but also the functionality of muscle tissue. This term encompasses both functional aspects, such as muscle strength and efficiency per unit of mass, and morphological factors, including muscle composition and architecture. Its significance goes beyond merely assessing muscle volume, offering crucial insights into health status, functional capacity, and the risk of chronic health conditions and disabilities, particularly among aging populations. However, despite its importance, there is considerable heterogeneity in how muscle quality is defined and evaluated in the scientific literature (Straight, Brady, and Evans 2015).

Different studies employ a variety of indices and evaluation methods, highlighting the complexity and multifaceted nature of muscle tissue (Heymsfield et al. 2015; Barbat-Artigas et al. 2013; McGregor, Cameron-Smith, and Poppitt 2014a; da Cunha Nascimento et al. 2020). This diversity, as revealed by various studies, underscores the urgent need for standardization in the definition and measurement of muscle quality. Such standardization would enhance the comparability of studies, facilitate the interpretation of results, and ultimately improve the design of interventions aimed at optimizing muscle health throughout life.

Muscle quality is conceptualized through two primary domains: functional and morphological (Figure 9.1). The functional domain focuses on the muscle's ability to generate force or power relative to its mass. This involves assessments of specific muscle strength, such as the ratio of knee extension strength to leg lean mass, providing a measure of how efficiently a muscle can perform work. In contrast, the morphological domain examines the structural characteristics of the muscle, including tissue composition (e.g., the ratio of muscle to adipose tissue) and architectural features such as echo intensity, which can indicate the quality of the muscle tissue (Coronado-Zarco and Olascoaga-Gómez de León 2023).

With aging, the musculoskeletal system undergoes significant changes at both neurological and morphological levels. Neurologically, there is a

DOI: 10.4324/9781003425182-12

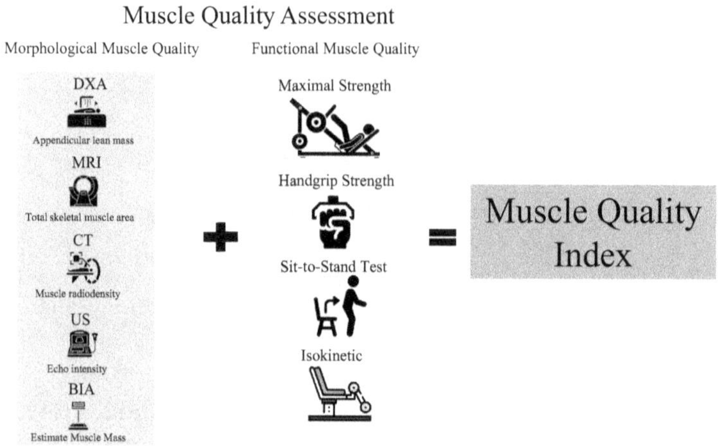

Figure 9.1 Instruments and key variables for evaluating muscle quality in its morphological and functional domains.

reduction in the number and efficiency of motor units, which directly impacts the muscle's ability to generate force. Morphologically, aging is associated with a decrease in muscle mass and changes in tissue composition, including an increase in the infiltration of adipose tissue within the muscle (myosteatosis). These changes not only lead to a reduction in muscle mass and strength (sarcopenia) but also deteriorate muscle quality, negatively affecting functionality, mobility, and independence in older adults (de Lucena Alves et al. 2023). Therefore, understanding and assessing muscle quality is crucial for identifying the risk of disability and developing effective strategies to maintain functionality and quality of life during aging.

Factors Influencing Muscle Quality

Several factors influence muscle quality in older adults, ranging from intrinsic biological processes to extrinsic lifestyle factors. These include the accumulation of intramuscular fat, changes in neural activation, metabolic health, physical activity, nutrition, hormonal fluctuations, and genetic predispositions (McGregor, Cameron-Smith, and Poppitt 2014a).

The accumulation of intramuscular fat (IMAT) and fibrous tissue, known as myosteatosis, is a critical factor in the decline of muscle quality. This condition leads to a reduction in both the contractile efficiency and metabolic capacity of the muscle fibers. Research indicates that older adults with elevated levels of IMAT exhibit less improvement in muscle quality following exercise interventions compared to those with lower IMAT levels (Marcus, Addison, and Lastayo 2013). Additionally, the increase in fibrous tissue within muscles decreases elasticity and strength, further exacerbating the decline in muscle quality with aging.

The aging leads to significant morphological changes in motor units, notably a decrease in the number of functional motor units. This reduction, where certain muscle fibers fail to undergo re-innervation, is expected to result in a decline in muscle quality. Moreover, age-related alterations in spinal properties and the neuromuscular junction—such as reduced spinal excitability and a decrease in maximal motor unit discharge rates—may further impair voluntary activation capacity, thereby contributing to the overall decline in muscle quality (Russ et al. 2012).

Metabolic health, particularly insulin sensitivity, is a crucial factor in maintaining muscle quality. The increase in insulin resistance associated with aging impairs glucose uptake and energy production within muscle cells, leading to decreased muscle functionality. Mitochondrial dysfunction, another age-related change, further reduces the muscle's capacity for energy production and management of oxidative stress. Chronic low-grade inflammation, prevalent in older adults, accelerates muscle degradation and increases intramuscular fat deposition, both of which negatively impact muscle quality (McGregor, Cameron-Smith, and Poppitt 2014b).

The Muscle Quality Index (MQI) in older adults is influenced by various factors (Kuschel, Sonnenburg, and Engel 2022). Age plays a significant role, with octogenarians showing lower MQI compared to younger older adults (Nascimento et al. 2020). Body composition, particularly BMI and diabetes mellitus, negatively affects MQI. Gender is also a factor, with women presenting lower MQI values than men (Jerez-Mayorga et al. 2020). Resistance exercise training can improve MQI in older adults (Fragala et al. 2014), while factors such as muscle composition, metabolism, and neural activation contribute to muscle quality beyond just muscle mass (McGregor, Cameron-Smith, and Poppitt 2014b). Obesity and muscle mass itself influence the relationship between MQI and physical function (S. Barbat-Artigas et al. 2012). Additionally, hip osteoarthritis is associated with lower MQI and reduced isometric strength in older adults (Jerez-Mayorga et al. 2019). These factors collectively impact muscle quality and its relationship with physical function in older populations.

Morphological and Functional Perspectives on Muscle Quality

In clinical practice, the absence of consensus regarding the definitions and assessment methodologies for muscle quality presents a significant challenge in utilizing muscle quality as a reliable outcome measure for both assessment and intervention. The proposed standardization, which encompasses specific domains (functional and morphological), terminology, and evaluation methods, offers a framework that can enhance the precision with which clinicians assess muscle quality and monitor the efficacy of interventions aimed at improving muscle health in older adults. For instance, the functional domain could be operationalized through the ratio of muscle strength—assessed via methodologies such as the one-repetition maximum (1-RM) test or isokinetic dynamometry—to muscle mass, measured by techniques like dual-energy X-ray absorptiometry (DXA), computed tomography (CT), magnetic resonance imaging (MRI), or bioelectrical impedance analysis (BIA). Emphasis on the quadriceps femoris is particularly pertinent, given its critical role in physical function and mobility, both of which are essential for preserving independence in older adults (de Lucena Alves et al. 2023).

Functional muscle quality encompasses the ability to generate force capable of altering the movement of an object, considering both the magnitude and direction of that force. This concept includes metrics such as relative strength, which is the ratio of peak force to body size or muscle area, and specific strength, which standardizes strength relative to muscle size (Table 9.1). Morphological assessments often involve parameters like fascicle length, muscle and tendon stiffness, muscle contraction characteristics, microcirculation, pennation angle, and echogenicity (Coronado-Zarco and Olascoaga-Gómez de León 2023) (Table 9.2). For a comprehensive evaluation, the integration of morphological and functional muscle quality is crucial. Techniques such as magnetic resonance imaging (MRI), computed tomography (CT), and ultrasound are employed to assess muscle composition, including fat infiltration (myosteatosis) and fibrosis, as well as muscle mass and volume. Lean mass can be measured through densitometry or bioimpedance, while cross-sectional area is commonly evaluated using MRI, CT, and ultrasound. In both clinical practice and research, it is vital to consider both morphological and functional muscle qualities for an accurate assessment of conditions like sarcopenia. Sarcopenia, defined by the age-related loss of muscle mass and strength, necessitates precise definitions and cut-off points for effective diagnosis and treatment. Therefore, assessing muscle quality should include the quantification of muscle performance factors such as power, strength, and work, in relation to muscle mass parameters like muscle thickness and physiological cross-sectional area.

Handgrip Strength and Muscle Quality Assessment

Handgrip strength (HGS) has been widely studied as a potential indicator of overall muscle strength and health status. Several studies have found strong correlations between HGS and total-body muscle strength (Binns, Gray, and Glenn 2016; Vaidya and Nariya 2021), suggesting its utility as a convenient and cost-effective assessment tool. HGS has been associated with various health outcomes, including mortality, morbidity, and functional capacity (McGrath et al. 2020; Bohannon 2019). It has also been linked to physical attractiveness, psychological well-being, and sexual history (Sneade and Furnham 2016).

Table 9.1 Definition of the Muscle Quality Index in its functional domain

Definition	*Test*
Muscle quality index uses timed sit to stand, individual body mass, and leg length to calculate a power index reported in watts (W) (Fragala et al. 2014). Muscle quality index = ((leg length × 0.4) × body mass × gravity × 10)/ time sit-stand.	Time to complete five consecutive full chair rises from a seated (timed sit to stand) and leg length.
"The muscle quality index was estimated by Handgrip strength (HGS) divided by body mass index" (Caamaño-Navarrete et al. 2023)	A hydraulic hand dynamometer was used to determine HGS. The measure of each dominant and non-dominant arm was made in two attempts, and the best result from each was selected. The average scores achieved by the left and right hands were registered for data analysis. MQI was categorized as follows: Low-MQI $\leq$ 50th and High-MQI > 50th (50th MQI = 0.67
"MQI (kg/kg) was defined as the ration between combined HGS divided by ASM. ASM is defined as the sum of the lean mass of arms and legs" (Weng et al. 2023).	HGS was measured by a handgrip dynamometer. Participants who had no surgery and pain on either hand or wrist in the last 3 months can be eligible for the test. The grip test was performed in the standing position and participants were requested to squeeze the dynamometer as hard as possible. Each hand was tested three times, with 60 sec between each test. The highest measurement of the hand was used. Body composition data obtained from DXA scans included arm lean mass (kg) and leg lean mass (kg). It's worth noting that lean mass from DXA includes both non-bone and non-fat tissue.
"The total MQI was determined by dividing subjects' Total Strength, as determined by the sum of the 3 1RM exercises, by the FFM. The upper-limb muscle quality (ULMQ) was determined by dividing the maximum load lifted in the PC by the arms lean soft-tissue mass, while the lower-limb muscle quality (LLMQ) was determined by dividing the maximum load lifted in the knee extension by the legs lean soft-tissue mass" (Ribeiro et al. 2022)	Maximal dynamic strength was evaluated using the 1RM test assessed on the chest press (CP), knee extension (KE), and preacher curl (PC) exercises, performed in this exact order. Fat-free mass (FFM) and body fat (BF) were evaluated by a dual-energy X-ray absorptiometry (DXA) scan.

(*Continued*)

Table 9.1 (Continued)

Definition	*Test*
The MQI (was determined by the following formula: MQI = Total Strength 1RM/Total Body SMM here "Total Strength 1RM" stands for the sum of load in kg obtained in 1RM tests in CP, KE and PC, and "Total Body SMM" stands for the skeletal muscle mass in kg calculated using lean soft tissue values (Fragala, Kenny, and Kuchel 2015).	One-repetition maximum (1RM) tests in chest press (CP), knee extension (KE), and preacher curl (PC), assessment of lean soft tissue and fat mass by dual energy X-ray absorptiometry (DXA), measurement of resistance, reactance, and PhA by spectral bioelectrical impedance were performed.
We defined the muscle quality index as the knee extension torque divided by the quadriceps femoris muscle thickness (Nm/cm) (Yamada et al. 2017).	Knee extension assessment using an isokinetic dynamometer to evaluate muscle strength and performance, combined with B-mode ultrasound imaging to measure muscle thickness as an indicator of muscle mass.

Table 9.2 Definition of the Muscle Quality Index in its morphological domain

Definition	*Test*
Muscle quality was assessed by echo intensity (Watanabe et al. 2013).	B-mode US (echo intensity) in the rectus femoris
Muscle quality was examined by intramuscular adipose tissue content at the L3 level (Hamaguchi et al. 2019).	CT at the level of the third lumbar vertebra (L3)
The Intracellular water content/lean mass ratio (in mL/kg) is used as an indicator of muscle quality (Serra-Prat et al. 2020).	BIA (intracellular water content/lean mass ratio)
Phase angle was defined as proxy of index of overall muscle quality (Irisawa and Mizushima 2022).	BIA (phase angle) in total body
Extracellular water/intracellular water ratio and phase angle were used as indices of muscle quality (Tanaka et al. 2022).	BIA (extracellular water/intracellular and phase angle) in total body
Muscle quality refers to micro- and macroscopic changes in muscle architecture and composition" (Jing et al. 2021).	Skeletal muscle radiodensity and intermuscular adipose tissue as proxy of muscle quality. CT images (radiodensity) in 12th thorax (T12) vertebral level

However, some research cautions against assuming HGS as a direct proxy for overall muscle strength, noting only low to moderate agreement between HGS and knee extension strength across different age groups and health statuses (Yeung et al. 2018).

The study by Yeung et al. (2018) critically challenges the assumption that HGS can serve as a proxy for overall muscle strength. The authors argue that while HGS is easy to measure, it does not necessarily reflect the strength of other muscle groups. This is particularly important when considering that overall strength encompasses various muscle groups beyond the hands and forearms, such as the core, legs, and upper body. The study highlights that relying solely on HGS could lead to an incomplete or even misleading assessment of an individual's overall strength.

Similarly, Tieland et al. (2015) conducted a study focusing on resistance training and its effects on muscle strength. Their findings further question the validity of using HGS as a measure of overall strength. The study observed significant improvements in muscle strength in a resistance training group, but these gains were not adequately reflected in HGS measurements. This suggests that HGS may not capture the full extent of strength gains achieved through comprehensive training programs, especially those targeting large muscle groups.

On the other hand, some studies suggest that HGS could still be a useful indicator, albeit with limitations. McGrath et al. (2020) found that HGS is associated with a range of health outcomes and is correlated with the strength of other muscle groups. However, the authors caution that while there is a correlation, it is not strong enough to justify using HGS as a sole indicator of overall strength. The association patterns between HGS and other strength measures vary depending on the population studied, the specific strength tests used, and other factors such as age and sex.

Porto et al. (2019) also explored the relationship between grip strength and global muscle strength. Their findings indicate that while there is a strong correlation, grip strength is not comprehensive enough to represent overall strength, particularly in clinical settings where precise assessment is crucial. The study suggests that grip strength should be considered a part of a broader battery of tests when assessing overall muscle strength.

Bohannon (2008) provides a broader perspective by discussing the multidimensional nature of muscle strength. The study emphasizes that strength cannot be fully captured by a single measure like HGS. Different measures of strength are often correlated because they reflect underlying neuromuscular function, but this correlation does not imply that one measure can stand in for another. The author argues for a more nuanced approach, where HGS is one of several indicators used to assess muscle strength comprehensively.

This conceptual approach is crucial when considering populations with specific needs, such as older adults or patients undergoing rehabilitation. In these cases, a singular focus on HGS might overlook other critical aspects of strength that are vital for functional independence and quality of life.

The synthesis of these findings suggests that while HGS can provide useful information, it should not be relied upon in isolation to assess overall strength. Practitioners and researchers are encouraged to use HGS as part of a multidimensional assessment strategy that includes other measures of muscle strength, such as leg press, chest press, or functional tests like sit-to-stand.

Muscle Quality Assessment with Functional Electromechanical Dynamometry

Upper Muscle Quality Index Through Handgrip Strength in FEMD

Muscle quality indices provide valuable insights into the relationship between muscle strength and muscle mass, helping to assess the functional capacity of individuals. In the context of evaluating muscle quality, several specific indices have been defined, each targeting different regions of the body using a combination of HGS measurements and Dual-energy X-ray Absorptiometry (DXA)-derived appendicular lean mass (ALM) (Mehra et al. 2024). In the case of not having a DXA measurement, another measure of body composition such as BMI, body mass or fat free mass can be used (Nascimento et al. 2020; Neto et al. 2023).

Muscle Quality Index of the Right Arm

The Muscle Quality Index of the Right Arm (MQI_{RA}) is calculated by taking the highest HGS measurement of the right hand and dividing it by the DXA-derived ALM specific to the right arm. This ratio provides an indication of how effectively the muscle mass in the right arm is contributing to its strength.

Muscle Quality Index of the Left Arm

Similarly, the Muscle Quality Index of the Left Arm (MQI_{LA}) is determined by dividing the highest HGS recorded for the left hand by the DXA-derived ALM of the left arm. This metric mirrors the MQI_{RA} but is focused on the left side of the body, allowing for the assessment of muscle quality in the left arm.

Muscle Quality Index of Both Arms

To obtain a more comprehensive view of upper limb muscle quality, the Muscle Quality Index of Both Arms (MQI_{ARMS}) combines the HGS values from both the left and right hands. The sum of these grip strength measurements is then divided by the combined ALM of both the left and right arms. This index provides a bilateral perspective on arm muscle quality, reflecting the overall functionality of both arms together.

Total Muscle Quality Index

Expanding beyond just the arms, the Total Muscle Quality Index (MQI_{TOTAL}) integrates the strength and lean mass of both the upper and lower limbs. This index is calculated by summing the HGS of both hands and dividing it by the total DXA-derived ALM, which includes the ALM of the left and right arms as well as the left and right legs. MQI_{TOTAL} offers a holistic measure of muscle quality, considering the entire appendicular musculature.

Muscle Quality Index

Muscle quality is a key indicator of physical function and overall health, representing the efficiency of muscle mass in generating strength. Various indices have been developed to evaluate muscle quality both at the total body level and within specific regions, such as the upper and lower limbs (Ribeiro et al. 2022; Tsai, Cheng, and Liu 2022). This section outlines the methodologies used to calculate these indices, providing a detailed understanding of how they are derived and their significance in assessing muscle function.

Total Muscle Quality

Total Muscle Quality (TMQ) is a comprehensive measure that reflects the overall efficiency of an individual's muscle mass in generating strength. To assess TMQ, maximal dynamic strength is evaluated using the 1RM test. This test is performed sequentially across several key exercises, starting with the chest press (CP), followed by knee extension (KE), and concluding with the preacher curl (PC). The total strength is determined by summing the highest 1RM achieved in each of these exercises. TMQ is then calculated by dividing this total strength by the individual's fat-free mass.

An alternative method for calculating TMQ involves incorporating additional exercises to provide a broader assessment of muscle quality. In this approach, the TMQ is determined by summing the 1RM values from four exercises: chest press, seated row, leg curl, and leg press. The resulting total strength is then divided by the total lean body mass, providing a holistic measure of muscle quality that encompasses both upper and lower body musculature.

Upper Limb Muscle Quality Index

The Upper Limb Muscle Quality Index provides a targeted assessment of muscle efficiency in the arms. It is calculated by dividing the maximum load lifted in the preacher curl (PC) by the lean soft-tissue mass of the arms. This index specifically evaluates how effectively the arm muscles generate force relative to their size.

In addition to the preacher curl-based index, another measure of upper-body muscle quality (UMQ) can be derived by combining the 1RM results from the chest press and seated row exercises. The sum of these 1RM values is then divided by the combined lean mass of the upper body and trunk. This approach offers a broader view of UMQ, considering not just the arms but also the trunk muscles that contribute to overall upper-body strength.

Lower Limb Muscle Quality Index

The Lower Limb Muscle Quality Index focuses on the efficiency of the leg muscles. One way to calculate this index is by dividing the maximum load lifted in the knee extension exercise by the lean soft-tissue mass of the legs. This ratio highlights the functional capacity of the leg muscles in relation to their mass.

Another approach to assessing lower-body muscle quality (LMQ) involves summing the 1RM values from the leg curl and leg press exercises. The combined strength from these exercises is then divided by the lean mass of the lower body. This method provides a comprehensive evaluation of LMQ, accounting for both the anterior and posterior muscle groups in the legs.

Functional Muscle Quality Index

Functional Muscle Quality Index (F-MQI) is a critical measure that reflects the capacity of muscles to produce force during functional tasks. One effective way to evaluate this is through the 5-repetition sit-to-stand (5-STS) test, which assesses the functional force generated by the lower limbs. This section details the methodology used to perform the 5-STS test and explains how the F-MQI is calculated using advanced equipment and specific formulas.

The Five-Repetition Sit-to-Stand Test

The five-repetition sit-to-stand (5-STS) test is a widely used functional test that simulates everyday movements, providing valuable insight into lower limb strength and endurance. For this test, participants are seated on a rigid chair with a seat height of 40 cm. Their arms are crossed over their chest, and their hip, knee, and ankle joints are positioned at approximately 90 degrees. On the command of a countdown (3, 2, 1), participants are instructed to stand up as quickly as possible, performing the concentric phase of the movement. The test involves completing five consecutive repetitions of the sit-to-stand motion.

To enhance the assessment, the 5-STS test is performed on a functional electromechanical dynamometer, with an additional load equivalent to 5% of the participant's body weight (BW). The external load is calculated based on the participant's BW, typically ranging from 2 to 6 kg for the 5% BW condition.

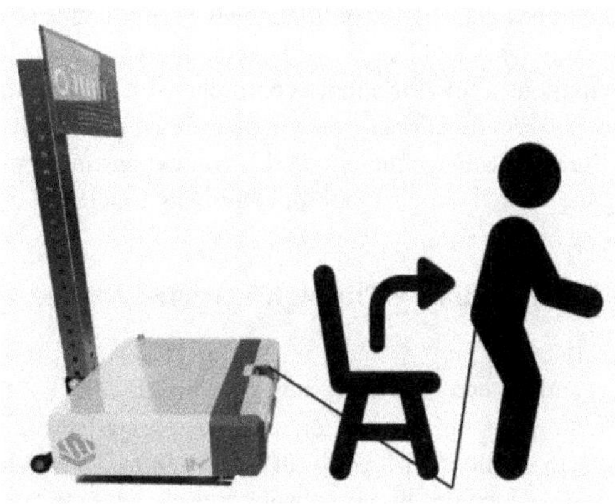

Figure 9.2 The five-repetition sit-to-stand (5-STS) test.

The FEMD is set to "Tonic Mode," which simulates the effect of a free weight, providing resistance throughout the motion. Peak force (measured in kilograms) is recorded during the concentric phase of each repetition using the FEMD's specialized software (Figure 9.2).

Calculation of the Functional Muscle Quality Index

Using the FEMD to accurately measure the force produced during the 5-STS test, two specific F-MQIs can be calculated. These indices provide a ratio of the peak force generated relative to different body composition metrics, offering a nuanced view of functional muscle quality.

F-MQI-FEMD Based on Lean Mass: This index is calculated by dividing the peak force recorded during the 5-STS test by the participant's lean mass (LM). The formula is as follows:

$$\text{F-MQI-FEMD} = \frac{\text{Peak Force in 5-STS}}{\text{Lean Mass (LM)}}.$$

This ratio provides insight into how effectively the participant's lean muscle mass contributes to functional strength during a fundamental movement pattern.

F-MQI-FEMD Based on Body Mass Index: Alternatively, the F-MQI can be calculated using the participant's body mass index (BMI) as the denominator. The formula is:

$$\text{F-MQI-FEMD} = \frac{\text{Peak Force in 5-STS}}{\text{Body Mass Index (BMI)}}.$$

This index offers a perspective on functional strength relative to the participant's overall body mass and height, as reflected in their BMI.

These calculations allow for a more comprehensive understanding of muscle quality by linking functional performance directly to body composition metrics. The use of FEMD technology in this context ensures precise measurement, making the F-MQI a robust tool for evaluating functional muscle quality.

Enhancing Muscle Quality Through Targeted Exercise Interventions

Exercise interventions can effectively improve muscle quality in older adults. Resistance training has emerged as one of the most effective strategies for improving muscle quality, particularly in older adults. Research consistently shows that resistance exercises can enhance muscle strength without a corresponding increase in muscle mass, leading to significant improvements in the muscle quality index. For instance, a study by Radaelli et al. demonstrated that resistance training significantly enhanced muscle strength and quality in older adults (Radaelli et al. 2021). This improvement is attributed to the neuromuscular adaptations that occur during resistance training, which enhance muscle function and efficiency.

Hortobágyi et al. further support these findings, showing that resistance training not only increases muscle strength but also improves neuromuscular function (Hortobágyi et al. 2023). These adaptations are crucial for older adults, as they contribute to better movement control and reduced risk of falls. The benefits of resistance training extend beyond just improving the MQI; they also include enhancements in bone density, metabolic health, and overall physical function, making it a cornerstone of exercise programs aimed at aging populations.

Resistance training has been shown to enhance both morphological and neuromuscular muscle quality, with small to moderate effects (Radaelli et al. 2021; Hortobágyi et al. 2023). Aerobic exercise also improves muscle quality, increasing myofibrillar protein synthesis and capillarization (Brightwell et al. 2019). Even short-term strength training programs of six weeks can significantly improve muscle quality and functional capacity in elderly women (Pinto et al. 2014). High-intensity stretch-shortening contractions have been proposed as an optimal exercise mode to combat age-related muscle decline (Baker 2018). Combined aerobic and strength training interventions have shown benefits for breast cancer survivors and healthy controls (Riley et al. 2021). Improvements in muscle quality are associated with enhanced muscle function, mobility, and overall physical performance (Fragala et al. 2014; McGregor, Cameron-Smith, and Poppitt 2014b). These findings suggest that various exercise modalities can effectively improve muscle quality in older adults, potentially mitigating age-related muscle deterioration.

References

Baker, Brent A. 2018. "Efficacy of Age-Specific High-Intensity Stretch-Shortening Contractions in Reversing Dynapenia, Sarcopenia, and Loss of Skeletal Muscle Quality." *Journal of Functional Morphology and Kinesiology* 3 (2). doi:10.3390/JFMK3020036.

Barbat-Artigas, Sébastien, Yves Rolland, Bruno Vellas, and Mylène Aubertin-Leheudre. 2013. "Muscle Quantity Is Not Synonymous with Muscle Quality." *Journal of the American Medical Directors Association* 14 (11). Elsevier Inc.: 852.e1–852.e7. doi:10.1016/j.jamda.2013.06.003.

Barbat-Artigas, Sébastien, Yves Rolland, M. Zamboni, and Mylène Aubertin-Leheudre. 2012. "How to Assess Functional Status: A New Muscle Quality Index." *The Journal of Nutrition, Health & Aging* 16 (1): 67–77. doi:10.1007/S12603-012-0004-5.

Binns, Ashley, Michelle Gray, and Jordan Glenn. 2016. "Hand-Grip Strength Relates to Total-Body Muscle Strength Among Older Adults." *Medicine & Science in Sports & Exercise* 48 (May). Ovid Technologies (Wolters Kluwer Health): 687. doi:10.1249/01.MSS.0000487063.51475.22.

Bohannon, Richard W. 2008. "Is It Legitimate to Characterize Muscle Strength Using a Limited Number of measures?" *Journal of Strength and Conditioning Research* 22 (1). NSCA National Strength and Conditioning Association: 166–173. doi:10.1519/JSC.0B013E31815F993D.

Bohannon, Richard W. 2019. "Grip Strength: An Indispensable Biomarker For Older Adults." *Clinical Interventions in Aging* 14. Dove Press: 1681. doi:10.2147/CIA.S194543.

Brightwell, Camille R., Melissa M. Markofski, Tatiana Moro, Christopher S. Fry, Craig Porter, Elena Volpi, and Blake B. Rasmussen. 2019. "Moderate-intensity Aerobic Exercise Improves Skeletal Muscle Quality in Older Adults." *Translational Sports Medicine* 2 (3). Wiley: 109. doi:10.1002/TSM2.70.

Coronado-Zarco, Roberto, and Andrea Olascoaga-Gómez de León. 2023. "Muscle Quality an Evolving Concept." *Journal of Frailty, Sarcopenia and Falls* 8 (4): 254–260. doi:10.22540/JFSF-08-254.

da Cunha Nascimento, Dahan, Jonato Prestes, Joyce de Sousa Diniz, Pedro Rodrigues Beal, Vicente Paulo Alves, Whitley Stone, and Fabiani Lage Rodrigues Beal. 2020. "Comparison of Field- and Laboratory-Based Estimates of Muscle Quality Index between Octogenarians and Young Older Adults: An Observational Study." *Journal of Exercise Rehabilitation* 16 (5). Korean Society of Exercise Rehabilitation: 458–466. doi:10.12965/jer.2040668.334.

de Lucena Alves, Charles Phillipe, Samuel Brito de Almeida, Danielle Pessoa Lima, Pedro Braga Neto, Ana Lúcia Miranda, Todd Manini, Lara Vlietstra, et al. 2023. "Muscle Quality in Older Adults: A Scoping Review." *Journal of the American Medical Directors Association* 24 (4): 462–467.e12. doi:10.1016/J.JAMDA.2023.02.012.

Fragala, Maren S., Anne M. Kenny, and George A. Kuchel. 2015. "Muscle Quality in Aging: A Multi-Dimensional Approach to Muscle Functioning with Applications for Treatment." *Sports Medicine (Auckland, N.Z.)* 45 (5): 641–658. doi:10.1007/S40279-015-0305-Z.

Fragala, Maren S., David H. Fukuda, Jeffrey R. Stout, Jeremy R. Townsend, Nadia S. Emerson, Carleigh H. Boone, Kyle S. Beyer, Leonardo P. Oliveira, and Jay R. Hoffman. 2014. "Muscle Quality Index Improves with Resistance Exercise Training in Older Adults." Experimental Gerontology 53 (May): 1–6. doi:10.1016/J.EXGER.2014.01.027.

Hamaguchi, Yuhei, Toshimi Kaido, Shinya Okumura, Atsushi Kobayashi, Hisaya Shirai, Siyuan Yao, Shintaro Yagi, et al. 2019. "Preoperative Visceral Adiposity and Muscularity Predict Poor Outcomes after Hepatectomy for Hepatocellular Carcinoma." *Liver Cancer* 8 (2): 92–109. doi:10.1159/000488779.

Heymsfield, Steven B., M. Cristina Gonzalez, Jianhua Lu, Guang Jia, and Jolene Zheng. 2015. "Skeletal Muscle Mass and Quality: Evolution of Modern Measurement Concepts in the Context of Sarcopenia." In *Proceedings of the Nutrition Society*, 74:355–366. Cambridge University Press. doi:10.1017/S0029665115000129.

Hortobágyi, Tibor, Tomas Vetrovsky, Jennifer S. Brach, Martijn van Haren, Krystof Volesky, Regis Radaelli, Pedro Lopez, and Urs Granacher. 2023. "Effects of Exercise Training on Muscle Quality in Older Individuals: A Systematic Scoping Review with Meta-Analyses." *Sports Medicine—Open* 9 (1). doi:10.1186/S40798-023-00585-5.

Irisawa, Hiroshi, and Takashi Mizushima. 2022. "Assessment of Changes in Muscle Mass, Strength, and Quality and Activities of Daily Living in Elderly Stroke Patients." *International Journal of Rehabilitation Research. Internationale Zeitschrift Fur Rehabilitationsforschung. Revue Internationale De Recherches De Readaptation* 45 (2): 161. doi:10.1097/MRR.0000000000000523.

Jerez-Mayorga, Daniel, Pedro Delgado-Floody, Leonardo Intelangelo, Christian Campos-Jara, Leonidas Arias-Poblete, Juan García-Verazaluce, Amador Garcia-Ramos, and Luis Javier Chirosa. 2020. "Behavior of the Muscle Quality Index and Isometric Strength in Elderly Women." *Physiology & Behavior* 227 (December): 113145. doi:10.1016/j.physbeh.2020.113145.

Jerez-Mayorga, Daniel, L. J. C. Ríos, A. Reyes, P. Delgado-Floody, R. M. Payer, and I. M. G. Requena. 2019. "Muscle Quality Index and Isometric Strength in Older Adults with Hip Osteoarthritis." *PeerJ* 2019 (8). doi:10.7717/peerj.7471.

Jing, Xiaofan, Lingling Tan, Hongbo Fu, Ling Yang, and Ming Yang. 2021. "Associations of ADL Disability with Trunk Muscle Mass and Muscle Quality Indicators Measured by Opportunistic Chest Computed Tomography Imaging Among Older Inpatients." *Frontiers in Medicine* 8 (October). doi:10.3389/FMED.2021.743698.

Kuschel, Luciano Bruno, Dominik Sonnenburg, and Tilman Engel. 2022. "Factors of Muscle Quality and Determinants of Muscle Strength: A Systematic Literature Review." *Healthcare* 10 (10). Multidisciplinary Digital Publishing Institute (MDPI). doi:10.3390/HEALTHCARE10101937.

Marcus, Robin L., O. Addison, and Paul C. Lastayo. 2013. "Intramuscular Adipose Tissue Attenuates Gains in Muscle Quality in Older Adults at High Risk for Falling. A Brief Report." *The Journal of Nutrition, Health & Aging* 17 (3): 215–218. doi:10.1007/S12603-012-0377-5.

McGrath, Ryan, Nathaniel Johnson, Lukus Klawitter, Sean Mahoney, Kara Trautman, Caroline Carlson, Ella Rockstad, and Kyle J. Hackney. 2020. "What Are the Association Patterns between Handgrip Strength and Adverse Health Conditions? A Topical Review." *SAGE Open Medicine* 8. SAGE Publications Ltd. doi:10.1177/2050312120910358.

McGregor, Robin A., David Cameron-Smith, and Sally D. Poppitt. 2014a. "It Is Not Just Muscle Mass: A Review of Muscle Quality, Composition and Metabolism during Ageing as Determinants of Muscle Function and Mobility in Later Life." *Longevity and Healthspan*. BioMed Central Ltd. doi:10.1186/2046-2395-3-9.

McGregor, Robin A., David Cameron-Smith, and Sally D. Poppitt. 2014b. "It Is Not Just Muscle Mass: A Review of Muscle Quality, Composition and Metabolism during Ageing as Determinants of Muscle Function and Mobility in Later Life." *Longevity & Healthspan* 3 (1). doi:10.1186/2046-2395-3-9.

Mehra, Ayush, Ronald L. Snarr, Kyung Shin Park, Jessica L. Krok-Schoen, Stefan A. Czerwinski, and Brett S. Nickerson. 2024. "Muscle Quality Index Comparisons between Hispanics and Non-Hispanic Caucasians Using Dual Energy X-Ray Absorptiometry and Handgrip Strength." *European Journal of Clinical Nutrition*. doi:10.1038/S41430-024-01484-Y.

Nascimento, Dahan da Cunha, Jonato Prestes, Joyce de Sousa Diniz, Pedro Rodrigues Beal, Vicente Paulo Alves, Whitley Stone, and Fabiani Lage Rodrigues Beal. 2020. "Comparison of Field- and Laboratory-Based Estimates of Muscle Quality Index between Octogenarians and Young Older Adults: An Observational Study." *Journal of Exercise Rehabilitation* 16 (5). Korean Society of Exercise Rehabilitation: 458–466. doi:10.12965/jer.2040668.334.

Neto, Ivo Vieira de Sousa, Joyce de Sousa Diniz, Vicente Paulo Alves, Alessandra Ribeiro Ventura Oliveira, Monica Palermo de Souza Barbosa, Carla Regina da Silva Prado, Jaqueline Alves Alencar, et al. 2023. "Field-Based Estimates of Muscle Quality Index Determine Timed-Up-and-Go Test Performance in Obese Older Women." *Clinical Interventions in Aging* 18: 293–303. doi:10.2147/CIA.S399827.

Pinto, Ronei Silveira, Cleiton Silva Correa, Regis Radaelli, Eduardo Lusa Cadore, Lee E. Brown, and Martim Bottaro. 2014. "Short-Term Strength Training Improves Muscle Quality and Functional Capacity of Elderly Women." *Age* 36 (1). Springer: 365. doi:10.1007/S11357-013-9567-2.

Porto, Jaqueline Mello, Ana Paula Midori Nakaishi, Luciana Mendes Cangussu-Oliveira, Renato Campos Freire Júnior, Sállua Berlanga Spilla, and Daniela Cristina Carvalho de Abreu. 2019. "Relationship between Grip Strength and Global Muscle Strength in Community-Dwelling Older People." *Archives of Gerontology and Geriatrics* 82 (May): 273–278. doi:10.1016/J.ARCHGER.2019.03.005.

Radaelli, Régis, Dennis R. Taaffe, Robert U. Newton, Daniel A. Galvão, and Pedro Lopez. 2021. "Exercise Effects on Muscle Quality in Older Adults: A Systematic Review and Meta-Analysis." *Scientific Reports* 11 (1). Nature Publishing Group: 1–11. doi:10.1038/s41598-021-00600-3.

Ribeiro, Alex S., Alexandre Picoloto, João Pedro Nunes, Ewertton S. Bezerra, Brad J. Schoenfeld, and Edilson S. Cyrino. 2022. "Effects of Different Resistance Training Loads on the Muscle Quality Index in Older

Women." *Journal of Strength and Conditioning Research* 36 (5). NSCA National Strength and Conditioning Association: 1445–1449. doi:10.1519/JSC.0000000000003667.

Riley, Sasha, Jordan T. Lee, Chad W. Wagoner, Kirsten A. Nyrop, Brian C. Jensen, Hyman B. Muss, Erik D. Hanson, and Claudio L. Battaglini. 2021. "16-Week Combined Exercise Training Improves Muscle Quality In Breast Cancer Survivors." *Medicine & Science in Sports & Exercise* 53 (8S). Ovid Technologies (Wolters Kluwer Health): 477–477. doi:10.1249/01.MSS.0000764836.89642.95.

Russ, David W., Kimberly Gregg-Cornell, Matthew J. Conaway, and Brian C. Clark. 2012. "Evolving Concepts on the Age-Related Changes in 'Muscle Quality'." *Journal of Cachexia, Sarcopenia and Muscle* 3 (2). Wiley Online Library: 95–109. doi:10.1007/S13539-011-0054-2.

Serra-Prat, Mateu, Isabel Lorenzo, Mònica Papiol, Elisabet Palomera, Maria Bartolomé, Eulogio Pleguezuelos, and Emili Burdoy. 2020. "Intracellular Water Content in Lean Mass as an Indicator of Muscle Quality in an Older Obese Population." *Journal of Clinical Medicine* 9 (5). doi:10.3390/JCM9051580.

Sneade, Michael, and Adrian Furnham. 2016. "Hand Grip Strength and Self-Perceptions of Physical Attractiveness and Psychological Well-Being." *Evolutionary Psychological Science* 2 (2). Springer Nature: 123–128. doi:10.1007/S40806-016-0042-Z/TABLES/3.

Straight, Chad R., Anne O. Brady, and Ellen M. Evans. 2015. "Muscle Quality in Older Adults: What Are the Health Implications?" *American Journal of Lifestyle Medicine*. SAGE Publications Inc. doi:10.1177/1559827613510681.

Tanaka, Hiroki, Gakuto Kitamura, Manabu Nankaku, Masashi Taniguchi, Kenichiro Shide, Miharu Fujita, Megumi Ida, et al. 2022. "Association of Physical Activity and Nutritional Intake with Muscle Quantity and Quality Changes in Acute Stroke Patients." *Journal of Stroke and Cerebrovascular Diseases: The Official Journal of National Stroke Association* 31 (6). doi:10.1016/J.JSTROKECEREBROVASDIS.2022.106442.

Tieland, Michael, Lex B. Verdijk, Lisette C. P. G. M. De Groot, and Luc J. C. Van Loon. 2015. "Handgrip Strength Does Not Represent an Appropriate Measure to Evaluate Changes in Muscle Strength during an Exercise Intervention Program in Frail Older People." *International Journal of Sport Nutrition and Exercise Metabolism* 25 (1): 27–36. doi:10.1123/IJSNEM.2013-0123.

Tsai, Shun Hsi, Hao Chien Cheng, and Hung Wen Liu. 2022. "Supervised High-Load Resistance Training for Improving Muscle Strength and Quality in Prediabetic Older Adults: A Pilot Randomized Controlled Trial." *Geriatric Nursing* 48 (November). Mosby: 350–355. doi:10.1016/J.GERINURSE.2022.11.001.

Vaidya, Shlesha Maulik, and Darshana M. Nariya. 2021. "Handgrip Strength as a Predictor of Muscular Strength and Endurance: A Cross-Sectional Study." *Journal of Clinical and Diagnostic Research*. JCDR Research and Publications. doi:10.7860/JCDR/2021/45573.14437.

Watanabe, Yuya, Yosuke Yamada, Yoshihiro Fukumoto, Tatsuro Ishihara, Keiichi Yokoyama, Tsukasa Yoshida, Motoko Miyake, Emi Yamagata, and Misaka Kimura. 2013. "Echo Intensity Obtained from Ultrasonography

Images Reflecting Muscle Strength in Elderly Men." *Clinical Interventions in Aging* 8: 993–998. doi:10.2147/CIA.S47263.

Weng, Luoqi, Zhixiao Xu, Yuhan Chen, and Chengshui Chen. 2023. "Associations between the Muscle Quality Index and Adult Lung Functions from NHANES 2011–2012." *Frontiers in Public Health* 11 (May): 1146456. doi:10.3389/FPUBH.2023.1146456/BIBTEX.

Yamada, Minoru, Yosuke Kimura, Daisuke Ishiyama, Naohito Nishio, Yuki Abe, Tomohiro Kakehi, Junko Fujimoto, et al. 2017. "Differential Characteristics of Skeletal Muscle in Community-Dwelling Older Adults." *Journal of the American Medical Directors Association* 18 (9): 807.e9–807.e16. doi:10.1016/J.JAMDA.2017.05.011.

Yeung, Suey S. Y., Esmee M. Reijnierse, Marijke C. Trappenburg, Jean Yves Hogrel, Jamie S. McPhee, Mathew Piasecki, Sarianna Sipila, et al. 2018. "Handgrip Strength Cannot Be Assumed a Proxy for Overall Muscle Strength." *Journal of the American Medical Directors Association* 19 (8). Elsevier: 703–709. doi:10.1016/J.JAMDA.2018.04.019.

10 Training Programs for Health and Quality of Life

Daniel Jerez-Mayorga and Daniel Jiménez-Lupión

Osteosarcopenia

Osteosarcopenia is a complex clinical condition characterized by the concurrent presence of osteoporosis and sarcopenia (Karacan and Türker 2024). Osteoporosis refers to the progressive loss of bone mass and deterioration of bone microarchitecture, leading to increased fragility and susceptibility to fractures. Sarcopenia, on the other hand, is the loss of skeletal muscle mass and function, which is strongly associated with increased risk of falls, frailty, and overall mortality in older adults. The coexistence of these two conditions significantly amplifies the risk of disability, loss of independence, and poor quality of life in the elderly population.

Age-related degenerative changes in nerve fibers that innervate bone and muscle tissues can disrupt the delicate balance of neuro-musculoskeletal interactions, contributing to the development and progression of osteosarcopenia. For instance, the decline in nerve fiber activity, reduced neurotransmitter release, and the loss of motor neurons are all factors that can lead to impaired muscle function and decreased bone strength (Allen et al. 2021).

The aging process also affects the mechanosensation capabilities of osteocytes. These cells, which are crucial for detecting mechanical loads and initiating appropriate biological responses, become less responsive with age. The structural integrity of the osteocytic network deteriorates, leading to impaired mechanotransduction and a reduced ability to maintain bone homeostasis (Choi et al. 2022). This decline in osteocyte function is a key factor in the development of osteoporosis and, consequently, osteosarcopenia.

Effects of Strength Training on Osteosarcopenia

Strength training, particularly high-intensity resistance training (HI-RT), has shown significant benefits in combating osteosarcopenia in older adults (Figure 10.1).

Multiple studies have demonstrated improvements in muscle mass, strength, and quality (Lichtenberg et al. 2019; Kemmler et al. 2020; Yang et al. 2022).

DOI: 10.4324/9781003425182-13

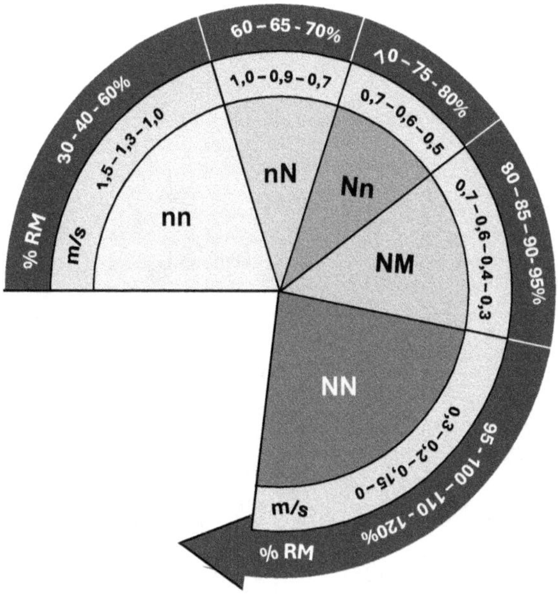

Figure 10.1 A proposed resistance training prescription for older adults with osteosarcopenia.

HI-RT has also been found to increase or maintain bone mineral density (Atlihan, Kirk, and Duque 2021; Kemmler et al. 2020) and reduce intermuscular adipose tissue (Ghasemikaram et al. 2021). The effectiveness of resistance training (RT) is supported by evidence showing improvements in sarcopenia Z-scores and physical function measures (Cunha et al. 2018; Lichtenberg et al. 2019). Additionally, RT has been found to be safe and well-tolerated in older populations (Roth, Ferrell, and Hurley 2000). Some studies have also explored the potential benefits of combining RT with nutritional interventions, such as protein supplementation, to enhance its effects on osteosarcopenia (Kemmler et al. 2020; Ghasemikaram et al. 2021) (Table 10.1).

The Role of Resistance Training in Mitigating Sarcopenia and Enhancing Health Across the Lifespan

While the decline in muscle function and structure associated with aging is inevitable, a multi-faceted approach involving exercise, proper nutrition, and pharmacological treatment can help prevent and slow the progression of sarcopenia and frailty (Yin et al. 2019; Sato et al. 2024). To date, it is widely recognized that physical exercise is a fundamental component in both the prevention

Table 10.1 Resistance training protocol

Study	*Means of intervention*	*Description*	*Time (min)*	*Frequency (times/week)*	*Period (weeks)*
(Cunha et al. 2018)	RT	The resistance training (RT) program followed a specific exercise sequence: chest press, horizontal leg press, seated row, knee extension, preacher curl (using free weights), leg curl, triceps push-down, and seated calf raise. Participants were divided into two groups, G1S and G3S. The G1S group performed one set of 10–15 repetitions to failure for each exercise, while the G3S group completed three sets of 10–15 repetitions to failure, with a one to two minutes rest between sets. Both groups trained until they could no longer maintain proper form. Participants were guided to inhale during the eccentric phase and exhale during the concentric phase, ensuring a controlled movement with a 1:2 second ratio for concentric and eccentric phases. The rest interval between exercises was two to three minutes. Progression was based on completing the upper limit of the repetition range for two consecutive sessions, after which the weight was increased by 2%–5% for upper limb exercises and 5%–10% for lower limb exercises (American College of Sports Medicine, 2009).	G1:30 G2: 50	3	12
(Ghasemikaram et al. 2021)	HIRT	The study implemented a periodized High-Intensity Resistance Training (HIRT) program, characterized by single-set exercise training with high effort. The training focused exclusively on intense resistance exercises performed on machines, targeting all major and minor muscle groups without incorporating other forms of exercise or warm-ups. Exercise intensity was managed by prescribing specific repetition ranges (e.g., five to seven or eight to ten reps) and monitoring the effort level. The program employed a classification system for set endpoints, including "non-repetition maximum" (nRM), "(self-determined) repetition maximum" (RM), and, in later stages, "complete momentary muscular failure." To quantify relative intensity (% 1RM) and effort, participants regularly performed 1RM tests for leg and bench presses. The 18-month intervention was divided into five mesocycles, each with distinct goals and protocols: First Period: Focused on education and selecting appropriate loads. Participants performed eight exercises as single sets and four exercises as double sets, with 8–15 repetitions per set and 90–120 seconds of rest. Second Period: Involved single sets of 14 exercises with 90 seconds of rest, using the Repetition in Reserve (RIR) approach. Third Period: Introduced the RM approach, with approximately one-third of sets including explosive concentric movements. Fourth Period: Incorporated a superset approach, targeting the same or related muscle groups (e.g., knee extension and leg press) or agonist and antagonist muscles (e.g., leg press and leg curls). Final Period: Added drop-sets, where after reaching RM (≤10 reps) or RM-1 rep, the load was reduced by 10%–20% to allow for additional repetitions, again to RM or RM-1 reps.	Not mentioned	2	64

(Continued)

Table 10.1 **(Continued)**

Study	*Means of intervention*	*Description*	*Time (min)*	*Frequency (times/week)*	*Period (weeks)*
(Lee et al. 2024)		Participants will undergo circuit RT using machines targeting major muscle groups, including four exercises for the lower extremities (leg press, leg abductor, leg flexor, leg extension), three for the upper extremities (chest press, row, dips), and one for core muscles (back extension). The training program is divided into three phases to progressively increase exercise intensity, with intensity determined using the non-repetition maximum (nRM) and repetition maximum (RM) methods. **Phase 1 (Weeks 1–8):** Participants will perform one to two sets of 8–15 repetitions using a self-determined weight that allows them to complete the prescribed range of repetitions (nRM: maximum effort minus one to three repetitions). Each repetition will follow a controlled tempo: two seconds for the concentric phase, one second for the isometric phase, and two seconds for the eccentric phase. Rest periods of 90–120 seconds will be allowed between sets or exercises. **Phase 2 (Weeks 9–16):** The intensity will be increased by adjusting the weight so that participants can perform seven to ten repetitions (nRM: maximum effort minus one repetition). The movement tempo will also be slowed to four seconds for the concentric phase, one second for the isometric phase, and four seconds for the eccentric phase, while maintaining the same rest intervals and exercise structure as in Phase 1. **Phase 3:** Participants will implement the RM approach, where they perform 7–10 repetitions to the point of momentary muscular failure (RM). To manage the increased intensity, a periodization strategy will be used, alternating three weeks of high-intensity exercise (RM) with one week of moderate-intensity exercise (nRM, as in Phase 1).	60	2	24

and management of sarcopenia (Cruz-Jentoft et al. 2019; Lauretani et al. 2014), and engaging in multicomponent exercise programs is currently recognized as an effective strategy for slowing the progression of sarcopenia and frailty (Paterson, Jones, and Rice 2007; Graham et al. 2021; Dent et al. 2023). Specifically, well-designed and closely monitored RT, aimed at preventing muscle atrophy and strength loss, has been recognized as the most effective and safe strategy for this purpose (Mcleod, Stokes, and Phillips 2019; Lavin et al. 2019; Cannataro et al. 2022; Zhao et al. 2022; Frontera et al. 1988). RT offers benefits such as preventing muscle loss, stimulating muscle growth, and preserving muscle function as we age, thereby mitigating the impact of sarcopenia (Sato et al. 2024).

RT is recommended for promoting health and preventing disease across all age groups (Muhu and Tilga 2023). Beyond just muscle hypertrophy and improved muscle function, regular RT provides a wide range of health benefits, including enhanced cardiovascular health (Paluch et al. 2024), better mobility and improved metabolic health (Weakley et al. 2023), increased bone density (Ponzano et al. 2021), cognitive function, and overall quality of life (Khodadad Kashi, Mirzazadeh, and Saatchian 2023). Additionally, RT is linked to a reduction in both all-cause and cancer-specific mortality (Burtscher, Millet, and Burtscher 2023). The World Health Organization recommends engaging in moderate-to-vigorous RT at least twice weekly (World Health Organization 2020).

Optimizing Resistance Training: Key Variables and Evidence-Based Protocols

RT prescription requires careful consideration of several key variables, including the load or resistance used (intensity), the number of sets (volume), training frequency, exercises order, and the contraction velocity (Bird, Tarpenning, and Marino 2005; Nunes et al. 2021). Currier et al. (2023) recently conducted a systematic review and Bayesian network meta-analysis to evaluate the impact of various RT protocols on muscle strength, hypertrophy, and physical function in healthy adults. This comprehensive analysis, which included data from 192 studies, offers a summary of the most current evidence gathered from nearly four decades of research. The authors examined 12 different RT protocols, considering combinations of load intensity (either lower or higher than 80% of one-repetition maximum (1RM)), sets (single or multiple), and weekly frequency (1×, 2×, or 3×+ sessions per week). The optimal approach identified was RT with higher loads, multiple sets, performed 2–3 times per week. However, all RT programs, whether involving lower or higher loads with more than three sets per exercise weekly, also resulted in significant improvements (Currier et al. 2023). Thus, understanding how different variables influence RT muscular adaptations is crucial for optimizing RT prescriptions and designing the most effective training programs tailored to everyone's specific characteristics and needs (Mcleod et al. 2024).

Resistance Training Intensity

During an RT program, individuals can use different loading zones ranging from 30% to 120% 1RM, which determine the training intensity (Figure 10.2). It has been suggested that combining different RT loading zones might produce synergistic effects on skeletal muscle adaptations (Schoenfeld et al. 2021). Studies evaluating the effectiveness of various training intensities have defined high-load as >75% of 1RM, moderate-load as 55%–75% of 1RM, and low-load as <55% of 1RM (Steib, Schoene, and Pfeifer 2010). Low-load RT (30%–50% of 1RM) can be as effective as higher-load training when performed close to failure (Weakley et al. 2023). However, using heavier loads has been a primary method for optimizing neuromuscular adaptations. Several systematic reviews provide ample evidence indicating that higher-load RT (≥80% RM) is crucial for maximizing gains in muscular strength (Lopez et al. 2021; Refalo et al. 2021; Schoenfeld et al. 2017). The advantage of higher-load RT for strength development is largely due to neural adaptations, such as increased neural

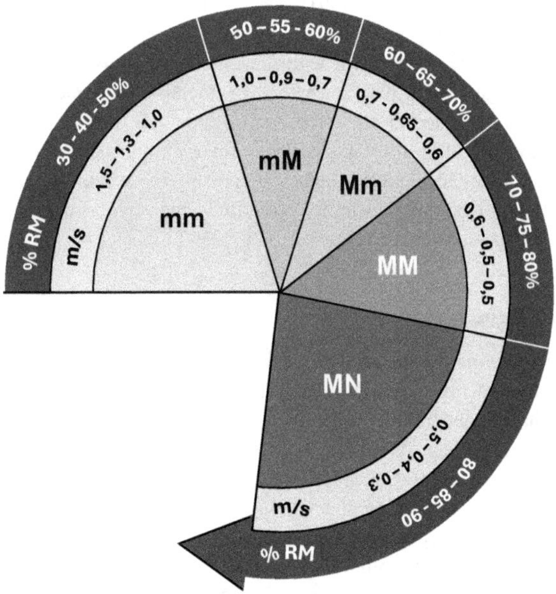

Figure 10.2 Resistance training load zones. For more details, see Chapter 4. Zones to Improve Different Expressions of Force.

drive, which occur when training with heavier relative loads (Jenkins et al. 2017). Guidelines suggest performing exercises targeting major muscle groups at moderate to high intensity (60%–80% 1RM) (Rhea et al. 2003; Fisher et al. 2011; Porter 2001).

Unlike strength gains, muscle hypertrophy appears to occur regardless of the RT load used when performed close to concentric failure (Weakley et al. 2023; Schoenfeld et al. 2017). Similarly, no significant differences have been observed between high-load and low-load RT in improving older adults' performance in stair climbing, timed up-and-go, chair rise, and walking speed tests (Steib, Schoene, and Pfeifer 2010). When the goal is to enhance functional capacity, variables such as movement velocity during the concentric phase of the movement appear to be more critical than load (Jiménez-Lupión et al. 2023).

The total work performed during RT is typically quantified by the number of sets completed in a single session or throughout a training week. The dose-response relationship between RT volume and skeletal muscle hypertrophy tends to follow an inverted-U pattern (Bernárdez-Vázquez et al., 2022; Schoenfeld et al., 2021). It has been shown that performing two to three sets per exercise and four to six sets per exercise resulted in greater hypertrophy than performing just one set per exercise. However, no significant difference in hypertrophy was observed between two to three sets per exercise and four to six sets per exercise (Krieger 2009). These findings suggest that while increasing RT volume initially provides additional hypertrophic benefits, there is a point of diminishing returns where further increases in volume yield progressively smaller gains and may even lead to negative outcomes. Therefore, it would be recommended to prescribe two to three sets of 6–15 repetitions per exercise, covering at least ten weekly sets for each muscle group (Rhea et al. 2003; Fisher et al. 2011; Porter 2001). Increasing the weekly volume beyond this threshold does not appear to provide further hypertrophy advantages (Bernárdez-Vázquez et al. 2022).

Resistance Training Frequency

Frequency is defined as the number of times a specific muscle group is trained in each period of time, usually a week (Schoenfeld et al., 2016). It has been observed that higher training frequencies (e.g., three days per week) provide a significant advantage for muscle hypertrophy when training volume is not equated across protocols (Schoenfeld et al., 2016). This may be because, when volume increases, increasing the weekly frequency allows maintaining the intensity of effort, thereby optimizing recovery between sessions. Instead, the authors found that when volume is equated, frequency does not significantly impact muscle hypertrophy. Therefore, for a given training volume, individuals can select a weekly training frequency for each muscle group based on their personal preferences (Schoenfeld et al., 2019). However, given that frequency is volume-dependent, increasing training frequency can be adjusted to allow for a higher total weekly volume, which has shown a dose-response relationship with hypertrophy (Bernárdez-Vázquez et al., 2022; Schoenfeld et al., 2021). Recommendations advise engaging in exercises that focus on the major muscle groups two to three times weekly (Rhea et al. 2003; Fisher et al. 2011; Porter 2001).

Exercise Selection and Order

For targeting specific muscle hypertrophy (e.g., triceps), some recommend performing single-joint exercises (e.g., triceps extensions) before multi-joint exercises (e.g., bench press) (Ribeiro et al. 2019). However, to maximize skeletal muscle hypertrophy during RT, it has been suggested that prioritizing multi-joint exercises over single-joint exercises could be beneficial due to the potential for greater training volume accumulation (Ratamess et al. 2009).

Regarding exercise order, it has been observed that dynamic strength gains were more pronounced in exercises performed at the beginning of an RT session, highlighting the principle of specificity. At the start of a session, individuals are less fatigued, allowing them to lift heavier loads and exert more effort (Nunes et al. 2021). Furthermore, findings from a recent umbrella review indicate that the order of exercises does not significantly affect hypertrophy outcomes, although it does impact strength gains (Mcleod et al. 2024). Therefore, to optimize maximal strength improvements and skeletal muscle hypertrophy, it is advisable to perform multi-joint exercises early in the training session.

Resistance Training in Older Adults

The fundamental principles of RT prescription apply to older adults as well. Training frequency is typically recommended at two to four sessions per week, with a sequence of three sets of 6–12 repetitions per exercise targeting major muscle groups (Rodrigues et al. 2022; Devries and Giangregorio 2023; Fragala et al. 2019). The intensity should range from 40% to 80% of 1RM, tailored to the individual's fitness level and health status. Training should be seen as a lifelong commitment. For beginners, it is advised to start with lower intensity in the first few weeks, gradually increasing it as tolerated. Rest periods of one to two minutes between sets are commonly recommended (Lopez et al. 2018).

An interesting variant of RT for older adults is known as power or velocity-specific training. This approach emphasizes fast concentric muscle actions paired with slow eccentric movements. This method is considered more functional because it incorporates "time" as a crucial factor, which is vital for performing many daily activities. In essence, many tasks in daily life, such as regaining balance to prevent a fall, require quick actions. The advantages of power or velocity-specific training for older adults have been confirmed in several clinical trials (Reid et al. 2008; Bean et al. 2009). Recent systematic reviews and meta-analysis also provided evidence that power training enhances both physical function and self-reported functional ability (Balachandran et al. 2022; Jiménez-Lupión et al. 2023).

Regarding power training intensity, a recommended range of 20% to 70% of 1RM is advised to optimize muscle power in the lower limbs (Izquierdo et al. 1999). However, research indicates that using low to moderate intensities (20% to 60% of 1RM) is equally effective in enhancing maximal strength, power output, functional capacity, and muscle mass in both healthy and frail older adults, including those with restricted mobility (i.e., scoring 8.1–8.8 on the short physical performance battery) (Cadore et al. 2014; Radaelli et al. 2018; De Vos et al. 2005; Reid et al. 2015; Izquierdo et al. 2021).

Proposal for Resistance Training Prescription for Healthy Adult Population

In summary, optimizing RT requires careful consideration of several key variables. Current evidence suggests using intensities ranging from 20% to 80% of 1RM, with a focus on higher loads to maximize muscle strength. It is advised to perform two to six sets of 6–15 repetitions per exercise, distributed across at least ten weekly sets per muscle group. The ideal training frequency is two to four times per week, prioritizing multi-joint exercises at the beginning of the session. Additionally, in power training for older adults, it is crucial to consider movement velocity, emphasizing fast concentric actions and slow eccentric phases. Rest periods between sets should be one to two minutes to allow for adequate recovery and maximize the benefits of the training session (Figure 10.3).

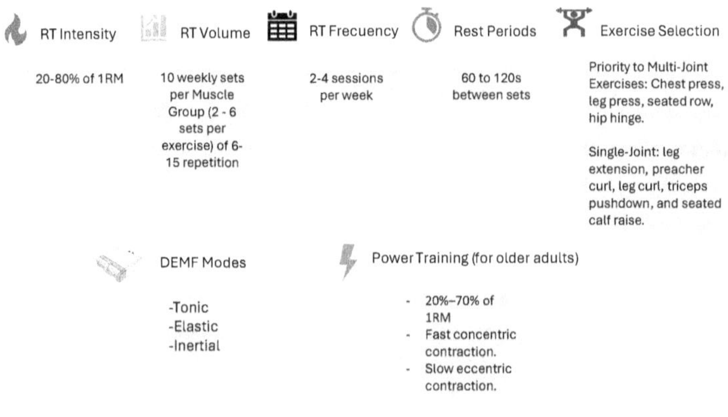

Figure 10.3 A proposed resistance training prescription for healthy adults.

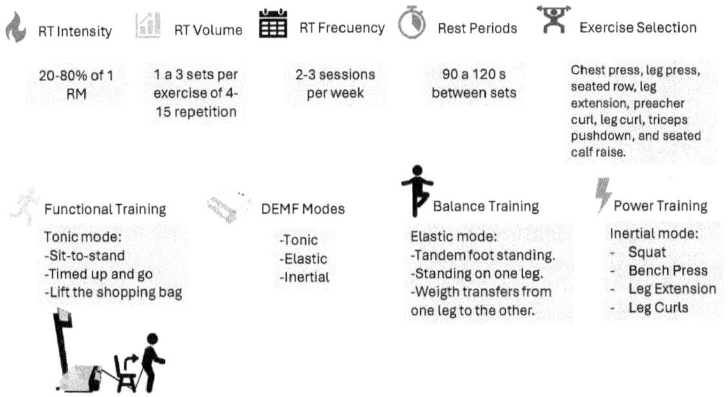

Figure 10.3 Continued.

References

Allen, Matti D., Brian H. Dalton, Kevin J. Gilmore, Chris J. McNeil, Timothy J. Doherty, Charles L. Rice, and Geoffrey A. Power. 2021. "Neuroprotective Effects of Exercise on the Aging Human Neuromuscular System." *Experimental Gerontology* 152 (September). doi:10.1016/J.EXGER.2021.111465.

Atlihan, R., B. Kirk, and Gustavo Duque. 2021. "Non-Pharmacological Interventions in Osteosarcopenia: A Systematic Review." *The Journal of Nutrition, Health and Aging* 25 (1). Elsevier: 25–32. doi:10.1007/S12603-020-1537-7.

Balachandran, Anoop T., James Steele, Daniel Angielczyk, Mark Belio, Brad J. Schoenfeld, Norberto Quiles, Nicole Askin, and Ahmed M. Abou-Setta. 2022. "Comparison of Power Training vs Traditional Strength Training on Physical Function in Older Adults: A Systematic Review and Meta-Analysis." *JAMA Network Open* 5 (5). American Medical Association: e2211623–e2211623.

Bean, Jonathan F., Dan K. Kiely, Sharon LaRose, Evelyn O'Neill, Richard Goldstein, and Walter R. Frontera. 2009. "Increased Velocity Exercise Specific to Task Training versus the National Institute on Aging's Strength Training Program: Changes in Limb Power and Mobility." *Journals of Gerontology Series A: Biomedical Sciences and Medical Sciences* 64 (9). Oxford University Press: 983–991.

Bernárdez-Vázquez, Roberto, Javier Raya-González, Daniel Castillo, and Marco Beato. 2022. "Resistance Training Variables for Optimization of Muscle Hypertrophy: An Umbrella Review." *Frontiers in Sports and Active Living* 4. Frontiers Media SA: 949021.

Bird, Stephen P., Kyle M. Tarpenning, and Frank E. Marino. 2005. "Designing Resistance Training Programmes to Enhance Muscular Fitness: A Review of the Acute Programme Variables." *Sports Medicine* 35. Springer: 841–851.

Burtscher, Johannes, Grégoire P. Millet, and Martin Burtscher. 2023. "Pushing the Limits of Strength Training." *American Journal of Preventive Medicine* 64 (1). Elsevier: 145–146.

Cadore, Eduardo L., Alvaro Casas-Herrero, Fabricio Zambom-Ferraresi, Fernando Idoate, Nora Millor, Marisol Gómez, Leocadio Rodriguez-Mañas, and Mikel Izquierdo. 2014. "Multicomponent Exercises Including Muscle Power Training Enhance Muscle Mass, Power Output, and Functional Outcomes in Institutionalized Frail Nonagenarians." *Age (Dordrecht, Netherlands)* 36 (2): 773–785. doi:10.1007/s11357-013-9586-z.

Cannataro, Roberto, Erika Cione, Diego A Bonilla, Giuseppe Cerullo, Fabrizio Angelini, and Giuseppe D'Antona. 2022. "Strength Training in Elderly: An Useful Tool against Sarcopenia." *Frontiers in Sports and Active Living* 4. Frontiers Media SA: 950949.

Choi, Jung Un Ally, Amanda W. Kijas, Jan Lauko, and Alan E. Rowan. 2022. "The Mechanosensory Role of Osteocytes and Implications for Bone Health and Disease States." *Frontiers in Cell and Developmental Biology* 9 (February). Frontiers Media S.A.: 770143. doi:10.3389/FCELL.2021.770143/BIBTEX.

Cruz-Jentoft, Alfonso J., Gülistan Bahat, Jürgen Bauer, Yves Boirie, Olivier Bruyère, Tommy Cederholm, Cyrus Cooper, et al. 2019. "Sarcopenia: Revised European Consensus on Definition and Diagnosis." *Age and Ageing* 48 (1). England: 16–31. doi:10.1093/ageing/afy169.

Cunha, Paolo M., Alex S. Ribeiro, Crisieli M. Tomeleri, Brad J. Schoenfeld, Analiza M. Silva, Mariana F. Souza, Matheus A. Nascimento, Luís B. Sardinha, and Edilson S. Cyrino. 2018. "The Effects of Resistance Training Volume on Osteosarcopenic Obesity in Older Women." *Journal of Sports Sciences* 36 (14). Routledge: 1564–1571. doi:10.1080/02640414.2017.1403413.

Currier, Brad S., Jonathan C. Mcleod, Laura Banfield, Joseph Beyene, Nicky J. Welton, Alysha C. D'Souza, Joshua A. J. Keogh, Lydia Lin, Giulia Coletta, and Antony Yang. 2023. "Resistance Training Prescription for Muscle Strength and Hypertrophy in Healthy Adults: A Systematic Review and Bayesian Network Meta-Analysis." *British Journal of Sports Medicine* 57 (18). BMJ Publishing Group Ltd and British Association of Sport and Exercise Medicine: 1211–1220.

De Vos, Nathan J., Nalin A. Singh, Dale A. Ross, Theodora M. Stavrinos, Rhonda Orr, and Maria A. Fiatarone Singh. 2005. "Optimal Load for Increasing Muscle Power during Explosive Resistance Training in Older Adults." *The Journals of Gerontology Series A: Biological Sciences and Medical Sciences* 60 (5). Oxford University Press: 638–647.

Dent, Elsa, Robin M. Daly, Emiel O. Hoogendijk, and David Scott. 2023. "Exercise to Prevent and Manage Frailty and Fragility Fractures." *Current Osteoporosis Reports* 21 (2). Springer: 205–215.

Devries, M. C., and L. Giangregorio. 2023. "Using the Specificity and Overload Principles to Prevent Sarcopenia, Falls and Fractures with Exercise." *Bone* 166. Elsevier: 116573.

Fisher, James, James Steele, Stewart Bruce-Low, and Dave Smith. 2011. "Evidence Based Resistance Training Recommendations." *Medicina Sportiva* 15 (3): 147–162.

Fragala, Maren S., Eduardo L. Cadore, Sandor Dorgo, Mikel Izquierdo, William J. Kraemer, Mark D. Peterson, and Eric D. Ryan. 2019. "Resistance

Training for Older Adults: Position Statement from the National Strength and Conditioning Association." *The Journal of Strength & Conditioning Research* 33 (8). LWW.

Frontera, Walter R., Carol N. Meredith, Kevin P. O'Reilly, Howard G. Knuttgen, and William J. Evans. 1988. "Strength Conditioning in Older Men: Skeletal Muscle Hypertrophy and Improved Function." *Journal of Applied Physiology* 64 (3): 1038–1044.

Ghasemikaram, Mansour, Oliver Chaudry, Armin M. Nagel, Michael Uder, Franz Jakob, Wolfgang Kemmler, Matthias Kohl, and Klaus Engelke. 2021. "Effects of 16 Months of High Intensity Resistance Training on Thigh Muscle Fat Infiltration in Elderly Men with Osteosarcopenia." *GeroScience* 43 (2). Springer Science and Business Media Deutschland GmbH: 607–617. doi:10.1007/S11357-020-00316-8/TABLES/3.

Graham, Zachary A., Kaleen M. Lavin, Samia M. O'Bryan, Anna E. Thalacker-Mercer, Thomas W. Buford, Kenneth M. Ford, Timothy J. Broderick, and Marcas M. Bamman. 2021. "Mechanisms of Exercise as a Preventative Measure to Muscle Wasting." *American Journal of Physiology. Cell Physiology* 321 (1): C40–C57. doi:10.1152/ajpcell.00056.2021.

Izquierdo, Ibañez, Gorostiaga, Garrues, Zúñiga, Antón, Larrión, and Häkkinen. 1999. "Maximal Strength and Power Characteristics in Isometric and Dynamic Actions of the Upper and Lower Extremities in Middle-aged and Older Men." *Acta Physiologica Scandinavica* 167 (1). Wiley Online Library: 57–68.

Izquierdo, Mikel, Olga Laosa, Eduardo L. Cadore, Pedro Abizanda, Francisco J. Garcia-Garcia, Mercedes Hornillos, Ignacio López-Pavón, Alan J. Sinclair, and Leocadio Rodríguez-Mañas. 2021. "Two-Year Follow-up of a Multimodal Intervention on Functional Capacity and Muscle Power in Frail Patients with Type 2 Diabetes." *Journal of the American Medical Directors Association* 22 (9). Elsevier: 1906–1911.

Jenkins, Nathaniel D. M., Amelia A. Miramonti, Ethan C. Hill, Cory M. Smith, Kristen C. Cochrane-Snyman, Terry J. Housh, and Joel T. Cramer. 2017. "Greater Neural Adaptations Following High-vs. Low-Load Resistance Training." *Frontiers in Physiology* 8. Frontiers Media SA: 331.

Jiménez-Lupión, Daniel, Luis Chirosa-Ríos, Darío Martínez-García, Manuel Rodríguez-Pérez, and Daniel Jerez-Mayorga. 2023. "Effects of Power Training on Functional Capacity Related to Fall Risk in Older Adults: A Systematic Review and Meta-Analysis." *Archives of Physical Medicine and Rehabilitation*, March. United States. doi:10.1016/j.apmr.2023.01.022.

Karacan, Ilhan, and Kemal Sıtkı Türker. 2024. "Exploring Neuronal Mechanisms of Osteosarcopenia in Older Adults." *The Journal of Physiology* 0. John Wiley & Sons, Ltd: 1–17. doi:10.1113/JP285666.

Kemmler, Wolfgang, Matthias Kohl, Franz Jakob, Klaus Engelke, and Simon von Stengel. 2020. "Effects of High Intensity Dynamic Resistance Exercise and Whey Protein Supplements on Osteosarcopenia in Older Men with Low Bone and Muscle Mass. Final Results of the Randomized Controlled FrOST Study." *Nutrients* 12 (8): 2341. Multidisciplinary Digital Publishing Institute: 2341. doi:10.3390/NU12082341.

Khodadad Kashi, Sholeh, Zahra Sadat Mirzazadeh, and Vahid Saatchian. 2023. "A Systematic Review and Meta-Analysis of Resistance Training on Quality of Life, Depression, Muscle Strength, and Functional Exercise Capacity in Older Adults Aged 60 Years or More." *Biological Research for Nursing* 25 (1). SAGE Publications Sage CA: Los Angeles, CA: 88–106.

Krieger, James W. 2009. "Single versus Multiple Sets of Resistance Exercise: A Meta-Regression." *The Journal of Strength & Conditioning Research* 23 (6). LWW: 1890–1901.

Lauretani, Fulvio, Ivan Bautmans, Francesca De Vita, Anna Nardelli, Gian Paolo Ceda, and Marcello Maggio. 2014. "Identification and Treatment of Older Persons with Sarcopenia." *The Aging Male* 17 (4). Taylor & Francis: 199–204.

Lavin, Kaleen M., Brandon M. Roberts, Christopher S. Fry, Tatiana Moro, Blake B. Rasmussen, and Marcas M. Bamman. 2019. "The Importance of Resistance Exercise Training to Combat Neuromuscular Aging." *Physiology (Bethesda, Md.)* 34 (2): 112–122. doi:10.1152/physiol.00044.2018.

Lee, Byung Chan, Kyung Il Kim, Kang Hee Cho, and Chang Won Moon. 2024. "Effects of Resistance Training and Nutritional Support on Osteosarcopenia in Older, Community-Dwelling Postmenopausal Korean Females (ERTO-K Study): A Study Protocol." *BMC Geriatrics* 24 (1). doi:10.1186/S12877-024-04667-1.

Lichtenberg, Theresa, Simon Von Stengel, Cornel Sieber, and Wolfgang Kemmler. 2019. "The Favorable Effects of a High-Intensity Resistance Training on Sarcopenia in Older Community-Dwelling Men with Osteosarcopenia: The Randomized Controlled FrOST Study." *Clinical Interventions in Aging* 14 (December). Dove Press: 2173–2186. doi:10.2147/CIA.S225618.

Lopez, Pedro, Ronei Silveira Pinto, Regis Radaelli, Anderson Rech, Rafael Grazioli, Mikel Izquierdo, and Eduardo Lusa Cadore. 2018. "Benefits of Resistance Training in Physically Frail Elderly: A Systematic Review." *Aging Clinical and Experimental Research* 30. Springer: 889–899.

Lopez, Pedro, Régis Radaelli, Dennis R. Taaffe, Robert U. Newton, Daniel A. Galvão, Gabriel S. Trajano, Juliana L. Teodoro, William J. Kraemer, Keijo Häkkinen, and Ronei S. Pinto. 2021. "Resistance Training Load Effects on Muscle Hypertrophy and Strength Gain: Systematic Review and Network Meta-Analysis." *Medicine and Science in Sports and Exercise* 53 (6). Wolters Kluwer Health: 1206.

Mcleod, Jonathan C., Brad S. Currier, Caroline V. Lowisz, and Stuart M. Phillips. 2024. "The Influence of Resistance Exercise Training Prescription Variables on Skeletal Muscle Mass, Strength, and Physical Function in Healthy Adults: An Umbrella Review." *Journal of Sport and Health Science* 13 (1). Elsevier: 47–60.

Mcleod, Jonathan C., Tanner Stokes, and Stuart M. Phillips. 2019. "Resistance Exercise Training as a Primary Countermeasure to Age-Related Chronic Disease." *Frontiers in Physiology* 10: 645. doi:10.3389/fphys.2019.00645.

Muhu, Andra, and Henri Tilga. 2023. "Strength Training Habits and Awareness of Its Recommendations among 18–63-Year-Old Adults." *Sustainability* 15 (6). Multidisciplinary Digital Publishing Institute: 5087.

Nunes, João Pedro, Jozo Grgic, Paolo M. Cunha, Alex S. Ribeiro, Brad J. Schoenfeld, Belmiro F. de Salles, and Edilson S. Cyrino. 2021. "What Influence

Does Resistance Exercise Order Have on Muscular Strength Gains and Muscle Hypertrophy? A Systematic Review and Meta-Analysis." *European Journal of Sport Science* 21 (2). Taylor & Francis: 149–157.

Paluch, Amanda E., William R. Boyer, Barry A. Franklin, Deepika Laddu, Felipe Lobelo, Duck-chul Lee, Mary M. McDermott, Damon L. Swift, Allison R. Webel, and Abbi Lane. 2024. "Resistance Exercise Training in Individuals with and without Cardiovascular Disease: 2023 Update: A Scientific Statement from the American Heart Association." *Circulation* 149 (3). Am Heart Assoc: e217–e231.

Paterson, Donald H., Gareth R. Jones, and Charles L. Rice. 2007. "[Aging and Physical Activity Data on Which to Base Recommendations for Exercise in Older Adults]." *Applied Physiology, Nutrition, and Metabolism = Physiologie appliquee, nutrition et metabolisme* 32 Suppl 2. Canada: S75–S171. doi:10.1139/H07-165.

Ponzano, Matteo, Isabel B. Rodrigues, Zeinab Hosseini, Maureen C. Ashe, Debra A. Butt, Philip D. Chilibeck, Jackie Stapleton, Lehana Thabane, John D. Wark, and Lora M. Giangregorio. 2021. "Progressive Resistance Training for Improving Health-Related Outcomes in People at Risk of Fracture: A Systematic Review and Meta-Analysis of Randomized Controlled Trials." *Physical Therapy* 101 (2). Oxford University Press: pzaa221.

Porter, Michelle M. 2001. "The Effects of Strength Training on Sarcopenia." *Canadian Journal of Applied Physiology* 26 (1). NRC Research Press Ottawa, Canada: 123–141.

Radaelli, Régis, Clarissa M. Brusco, Pedro Lopez, Anderson Rech, Carlos L. F. Machado, Rafael Grazioli, Diana C. Müller, Eduardo L. Cadore, and Ronei S. Pinto. 2018. "Higher Muscle Power Training Volume Is Not Determinant for the Magnitude of Neuromuscular Improvements in Elderly Women." *Experimental Gerontology* 110. Elsevier: 15–22.

Ratamess, Nicholas A., Brent A. Alvar, Tammy K. Evetoch, Terry J. Housh, W. Ben Kibler, William J. Kraemer, N. Travis Triplett, and American College of Sports Medicine. 2009. "Progression Models in Resistance Training for Healthy Adults." *Medicine & Science in Sports & Exercise: Official Journal of the American College of Sports Medicine* 41 (3). Lippincott Williams & Wilkins: 687–708.

Refalo, Martin C., D. Lee Hamilton, D. Robert Paval, Iain J. Gallagher, Simon A. Feros, and Jackson J. Fyfe. 2021. "Influence of Resistance Training Load on Measures of Skeletal Muscle Hypertrophy and Improvements in Maximal Strength and Neuromuscular Task Performance: A Systematic Review and Meta-Analysis." *Journal of Sports Sciences* 39 (15). Taylor & Francis: 1723–1745.

Reid, Kieran F., Damien M. Callahan, Robert J. Carabello, Edward M. Phillips, Walter R. Frontera, and Roger A. Fielding. 2008. "Lower Extremity Power Training in Elderly Subjects with Mobility Limitations: A Randomized Controlled Trial." *Aging Clinical and Experimental Research* 20. Springer: 337–343.

Reid, Kieran F., Kimberly I. Martin, Gheorghe Doros, David J. Clark, Cynthia Hau, Carolynn Patten, Edward M. Phillips, Walter R. Frontera, and Roger A. Fielding. 2015. "Comparative Effects of Light or Heavy Resistance Power

Training for Improving Lower Extremity Power and Physical Performance in Mobility-Limited Older Adults." *Journals of Gerontology Series A: Biomedical Sciences and Medical Sciences* 70 (3). Oxford University Press US: 374–380.

Rhea, Matthew R., Brent A. Alvar, Lee N. Burkett, and Stephen D. Ball. 2003. "A Meta-Analysis to Determine the Dose Response for Strength Development." *Medicine & Science in Sports & Exercise* 35 (3). LWW: 456–464.

Ribeiro, Alex S., Joao Pedro Nunes, Paolo M. Cunha, Andreo F. Aguiar, and Brad J. Schoenfeld. 2019. "Potential Role of Pre-Exhaustion Training in Maximizing Muscle Hypertrophy: A Review of the Literature." *Strength & Conditioning Journal* 41 (1). LWW: 75–80.

Rodrigues, Filipe, Christophe Domingos, Diogo Monteiro, and Pedro Morouço. 2022. "A Review on Aging, Sarcopenia, Falls, and Resistance Training in Community-Dwelling Older Adults." *International Journal of Environmental Research and Public Health* 19 (2). MDPI: 874.

Roth, S. M., R. E. Ferrell, and B. F. Hurley. 2000. "Strength Training for the Prevention and Treatment of Sarcopenia." *The Journal of Nutrition, Health & Aging* 4 (3). Springer-Verlag Italia s.r.l.: 143–155. doi:10.29199/boms.101015.

Sato, Ryosuke, Mirela Vatic, Guilherme Wesley Peixoto da Fonseca, Stefan D. Anker, and Stephan von Haehling. 2024. "Biological Basis and Treatment of Frailty and Sarcopenia." *Cardiovascular Research*, June. England. doi:10.1093/cvr/cvae073.

Schoenfeld, Brad Jon, James Fisher, Jozo Grgic, Cody Haun, Eric Helms, Stuart Phillips, James Steele, and Andrew Vigotsky. 2021. "Resistance Training Recommendations to Maximize Muscle Hypertrophy in an Athletic Population: Position Stand of the IUSCA." *International Journal of Strength and Conditioning* 1 (1).

Schoenfeld, Brad Jon, Jozo Grgic, and James Krieger. 2019. "How Many Times per Week Should a Muscle Be Trained to Maximize Muscle Hypertrophy? A Systematic Review and Meta-Analysis of Studies Examining the Effects of Resistance Training Frequency." *Journal of Sports Sciences* 37 (11). Taylor & Francis: 1286–1295.

Schoenfeld, Brad Jon, Jozo Grgic, Dan Ogborn, and James W. Krieger. 2017. "Strength and Hypertrophy Adaptations between Low-vs. High-Load Resistance Training: A Systematic Review and Meta-Analysis." *The Journal of Strength & Conditioning Research* 31 (12). LWW: 3508–3523.

Schoenfeld, Brad Jon, Dan Ogborn, and James W Krieger. 2016. "Effects of Resistance Training Frequency on Measures of Muscle Hypertrophy: A Systematic Review and Meta-Analysis." *Sports Medicine* 46 (11). Springer: 1689–1697.

Steib, Simon, Daniel Schoene, and Klaus Pfeifer. 2010. "Dose-Response Relationship of Resistance Training in Older Adults: A Meta-Analysis." *Medicine & Science in Sports & Exercise* 42 (5). LWW: 902–914.

Weakley, Jonathon, Brad J. Schoenfeld, Johanna Ljungberg, Shona L. Halson, and Stuart M. Phillips. 2023. "Physiological Responses and Adaptations to Lower Load Resistance Training: Implications for Health and Performance." *Sports Medicine-Open* 9 (1). Springer: 28.

World Health Organization. 2020. *WHO Guidelines on Physical Activity and Sedentary Behaviour*. World Health Organization.

Yang, Jia ming, Hua Ye, Qiang Zhu, Jia hong Zhang, Qin qin Liu, Hui yong Xie, Yi Long, et al. 2022. "Effects of Resistance Training on Body Composition and Physical Function in Elderly Patients with Osteosarcopenic Obesity: A Systematic Review and Meta-Analysis." *Archives of Osteoporosis* 17 (1). Springer Science and Business Media Deutschland GmbH: 1–11. doi:10.1007/S11657-022-01120-X/TABLES/3.

Yin, Jiayu, Xiang Lu, Zhiyuan Qian, Weiting Xu, and Xiang Zhou. 2019. "New Insights into the Pathogenesis and Treatment of Sarcopenia in Chronic Heart Failure." *Theranostics* 9 (14). Ivyspring International Publisher: 4019.

Zhao, Haotian, Ruihong Cheng, Ge Song, Jin Teng, Siqin Shen, Xuancheng Fu, Yi Yan, and Chang Liu. 2022. "The Effect of Resistance Training on the Rehabilitation of Elderly Patients with Sarcopenia: A Meta-Analysis." *International Journal of Environmental Research and Public Health* 19 (23). MDPI: 15491.

11 Musculoskeletal Injuries and Muscle Quality

Ángela Rodríguez-Perea and Darío Martínez-García

Low Back Pain

Low back pain (LBP) is one of the most recurrent musculoskeletal injuries in the population, being a leading cause of disability worldwide. It is anticipated that by the year 2050, 843 million people worldwide will suffer from LBP, representing a 36.4% increase compared to 2020. Additionally, it is estimated that 80% of the population currently suffers from or will experience LBP at some point in their lives. Therefore, it stands as one of the most significant health problems globally (Ferreira et al. 2023).

Ninety percent of LBP cases are not associated with any specific cause, with the onset of this pain being multifactorial. Among the various factors that may affect the onset of pain are age, weight, and sex (Ferreira et al. 2023; Calais-Ferreira et al. 2023; Fehrmann et al. 2019) (Figure 11.1); weakened lumbar or abdominal musculature, as well as reduced trunk muscle mass and strength (Hodges and Danneels 2019; Steele, Bruce-Low, and Smith 2014; Cho et al. 2014; Catalá et al. 2018; Hori et al. 2019). Additionally, other factors such as social influence and psychological aspects can impact this condition. Regarding the structure and muscular function of the trunk, extensive research has been conducted to understand its relationship with the onset of LBP. Recent studies have shown that the replacement of muscular tissue with non-contractile adipose tissue in the lumbar musculature leads to a decrease in functional capacity (Hamrick, McGee-Lawrence, and Frechette 2016; Zhu et al. 2023).

Therefore, it is necessary to assess the strength of the trunk musculature to understand the risk of experiencing LBP, as well as to determine the individual's functional status. Various methods exist for evaluating trunk strength, including laboratory tests and field tests. Within laboratory tests, there are numerous devices available for assessing trunk strength, such as isokinetic devices (Verbrugghe et al. 2019; García-Vaquero et al. 2020; Roth et al. 2017), handheld (De Blaiser et al. 2018), isoinertial dynamometers (Zemkova 2019; Zemková et al. 2017), load cells (Steeves et al. 2019; Mesquita et al. 2019), and functional electromechanical dynamometer (Reyes-Ferrada, Rodríguez-Perea, et al. 2022;

DOI: 10.4324/9781003425182-14

Rodriguez-Perea et al. 2019a). Regarding field tests, one of the most used are the Biering-Sorensen test (Shaw et al. 2023), the front plank test (Bohannon et al. 2018), the side plank test (Juan-Recio et al. 2017), the ito test (Juan-Recio et al. 2014), and 60-degree flexor endurance test (Juan-Recio et al. 2014).

All these tests assess the trunk musculature's capacity. In the case of laboratory tests, values such as strength, work, power, and force ratios can be obtained or calculated. In field tests, the value obtained is often the number of repetitions or the time a participant can maintain a position. Therefore, if we want to obtain strength values, it is important to assess trunk musculature with laboratory tests.

Isokinetic devices are considered the gold standard for assessing trunk musculature. Their validity and reliability for conducting these evaluations have been studied for many years, yielding very good results. However, these devices are expensive and challenging to use. An alternative to these devices is hand-held dynamometers, but they have a disadvantage: assessments can only be performed isometrically, like load cells.

On the other hand, FEMD allows for the assessment of trunk strength in all planes and modes of contraction. In the last five years, protocols have been developed to evaluate trunk musculature in healthy young individuals, which are then applied to subjects with LBP (Rodriguez-Perea et al. 2019b; Rodríguez-Perea et al. 2023; Reyes-Ferrada, Chirosa-Rios, et al. 2022). In an initial study, different velocities and ranges of motion were compared to determine the most reliable protocol for evaluating trunk flexor musculature. It was concluded that the lowest velocity (0.15 ms^{-1}) and the shortest range of motion (25%) are the most reliable conditions for assessing trunk flexors in a seated position using a functional electromechanical dynamometer (Rodriguez-Perea et al. 2019a). In a subsequent study, the same methodology was applied to evaluate trunk extensors, yielding similar results regarding the recommended evaluation protocol (Reyes-Ferrada, Chirosa-Rios, et al. 2022) (Figure 11.1).

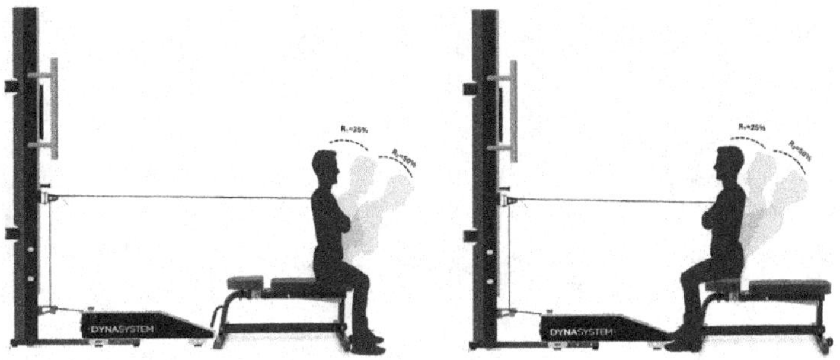

Figure 11.1 Set-up of trunk flexors and extensors assessment.

Upon determining that slow velocities and short ranges are the most reliable conditions for assessing healthy young individuals, a study was conducted to determine the reliability of evaluations in individuals with non-specific LBP. In trunk flexors, very high-reliability values were obtained (ICC > 0.87; CV < 13.64%) for concentric, eccentric, and isometric contractions, as well as for peak force and mean force variables. Similarly, in trunk extensors, similar values were obtained (ICC > 0.87; CV < 15.63%) (Figure 11.2).

Furthermore, in recent studies, the reliability of two exercises for measuring trunk rotator muscle strength was analyzed. The woodchop exercise was performed with both low pulley and horizontal pulley to compare reliability at slow and moderate speeds in healthy young individuals. Like the assessment of flexor and extensor trunk musculature, slower velocities were found to be more reliable. Besides comparing velocities, both exercises were compared, concluding that the woodchop exercise with a horizontal pulley is more reliable

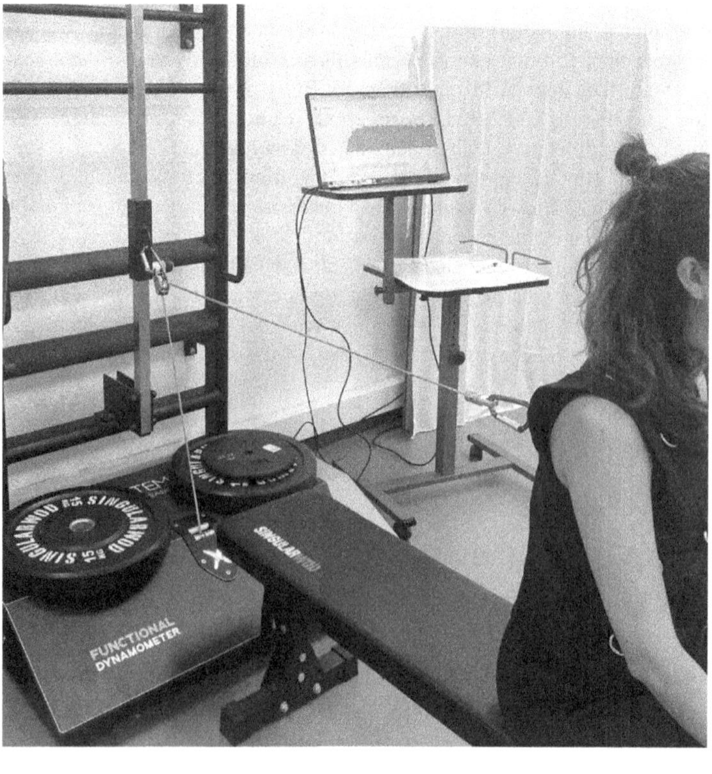

Figure 11.2 Isometric assessment of trunk flexors.

than with a low pulley (Rodríguez-Perea et al. 2023). Once the most reliable exercise and velocity were determined, individuals with non-specific LBP were evaluated, yielding very high reliability for both right-sided rotators (ICC > 0.91; CV < 10.10%) and left-sided rotators (ICC > 0.86; CV < 11.86%) for all types of contractions and with variables of mean force and peak force.

Musculoskeletal injuries, particularly low back pain, are closely linked to muscle quality.

- **Muscle Imbalance and Weakness:** Poor muscle quality, characterized by muscle weakness, atrophy, or imbalance, can lead to improper spinal alignment and increased strain on the lower back. Weak core muscles, especially the deep stabilizers like the multifidus and transversus abdominis, can fail to support the spine effectively, contributing to low back pain.
- **Fatty Infiltration and Degeneration:** Reduced muscle quality often involves fatty infiltration and degeneration of the lumbar muscles, particularly the lumbar multifidus and erector spinae. This can reduce muscle function and endurance, leading to chronic low back pain and impaired mobility.
- **Poor Muscle Activation:** Inadequate muscle activation patterns, often resulting from or contributing to poor muscle quality, can exacerbate stress on the lumbar spine during activities, further contributing to low back pain.

Shoulder Pain

The shoulder joint is integral to a wide array of daily live activities, serving as a pivotal point for the execution of movements involving the arms and upper body. Its unique anatomical structure allows for an extensive range of motion, making it one of the most mobile joints in the human body. This mobility allows people to do activities such as placing things on shelves, hammering, or carrying bags, among others. However, the shoulder's complexity and extensive range of motion also make it vulnerable to injuries (see Figure 11.3), particularly in activities that require repetitive overhead motions or direct impact (Kibler, Wilkes, and Sciascia 2013).

Shoulder injuries are a significant concern not only due to their frequency but also because of their impact on people's quality of life. These injuries can lead to substantial pain, decreased range of motion, and a prolonged period of recovery, often requiring both surgical intervention and extensive physical therapy. Studies indicate that shoulder injuries account for a considerable percentage of musculoskeletal injuries, with conditions such as rotator cuff tears, dislocations, and tendinitis being most common (Seitz and Haff 2016).

1. **Dislocations:** Shoulder dislocations occur when the head of the humerus is displaced from the glenoid fossa, often due to a sudden impact or extreme external rotation and abduction of the arm. This injury is common in contact

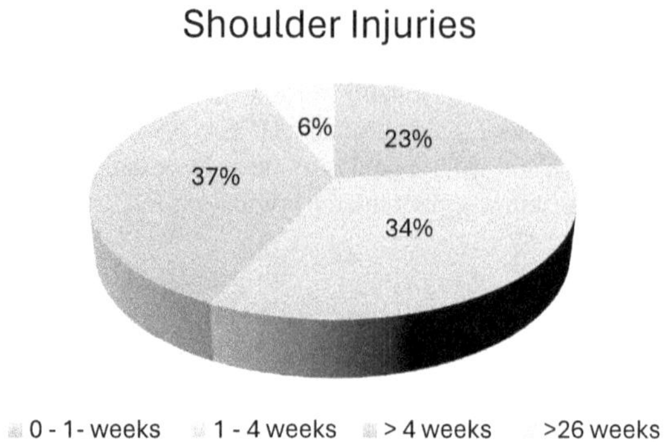

Figure 11.3 Shoulder injury incidence.

sports such as football and rugby and can lead to chronic instability if not properly addressed (Owens, Campbell, and Cameron 2013).

2. **Tendinitis:** Often resulting from overuse, tendinitis involves inflammation of the tendons of the rotator cuff. This condition is typical among athletes who engage in repetitive overhead activities, such as swimmers and baseball pitchers. Persistent stress can lead to micro-tears and degeneration of tendon tissue, exacerbating pain and functional impairment (Seitz et al. 2016).
3. **Rotator Cuff Tears:** These injuries range from partial to full thickness tears and are particularly debilitating. They occur due to acute trauma or progressive degeneration and can significantly impair shoulder function. Athletes involved in repetitive throwing or lifting activities are at higher risk for rotator cuff tears (Edwards et al. 2020).

Clinical evaluation of the shoulder is comprehensive and involves a variety of techniques designed to assess the structure and function of the shoulder complex. The assessment typically begins with a detailed patient history to understand the nature and mechanism of the injury. Physical examinations include visual inspection, palpation, range of motion (ROM) tests, strength tests, and specific orthopedic tests. These clinical evaluations are crucial for identifying the type and extent of injury and for guiding further diagnostic imaging or isokinetic testing (Whinton et al. 2018).

The *gold standard* for strength evaluation is isokinetic testing. These kinds of evaluations measure the strength and mechanical performance of muscles at a constant speed, regardless of the force applied. This method provides a dynamic assessment of muscle strength throughout the entire range of motion, distinguishing it from static measurements such as isometric testing (Andersen et al. 2014).

In the context of shoulder evaluation, isokinetic testing is particularly useful for quantifying the strength of the rotator cuff muscles and the muscles that stabilize the scapula. The common protocols involve assessing the concentric and eccentric contractions of the internal and external rotators and the flexors and extensors of the shoulder. This information is vital for identifying specific weaknesses that may predispose people to injuries or that may have developed as a result of injury. Isokinetic tests can be integrated into both the initial assessment phase and the rehabilitation process to monitor progress and the effectiveness of treatment strategies (Kibler, Wilkes, and Sciascia 2013).

Interpreting the results from isokinetic testing involves analyzing the data on muscle strength, endurance, and the balance between opposing muscle groups (such as the internal and external rotators). Key metrics from these tests include peak torque, total work, and the torque curve throughout the range of motion. It is also important to assess the symmetry between the injured and uninjured shoulders. Significant asymmetries can indicate areas of weakness or compensation, guiding the focus of rehabilitation. Clinicians use this data to tailor rehabilitation programs specifically to the athlete's needs, aiming to restore balance and function to the shoulder complex (Davies and Ellenbecker 2012).

In recent years, significant progress has been made in biomechanical assessment techniques enhancing our understanding and capability to diagnose and rehabilitate shoulder injuries effectively. A notable development in this area is the use of functional electromechanical dynamometers, which have shown promising results in the reliable assessment of shoulder function.

Some studies have explored various protocols for evaluating the shoulder musculature using FEMD. For instance, Martinez-Garcia et al. (2020) investigated different velocities and ranges of motion to determine the most reliable conditions for assessing shoulder rotator strength. Their findings indicated that lower velocities and shorter ranges of motion provided the most reliable assessments. This protocol adjustment is crucial for ensuring precision and repeatability in clinical evaluations, which are essential for both diagnosis and monitoring rehabilitation progress (Figure 11.4).

These studies highlighted that the reliability of shoulder strength assessments could be significantly enhanced by optimizing the test conditions. The researchers recommended a specific protocol involving slow velocities and minimal joint movement to reduce variability and improve the accuracy of the results. These protocols proved particularly effective for both concentric and eccentric contractions, which are critical for understanding the dynamic function of the shoulder movement.

The optimized protocol has been applied in various clinical settings, yielding highly reliable outcomes. For instance, assessments conducted under these controlled conditions showed very high reliability (ICC > 0.90; CV $< 10\%$) across different types of muscular contractions and strength measurements. This level of reliability is essential for developing targeted rehabilitation programs and tracking the recovery of athletes or patients with shoulder injuries.

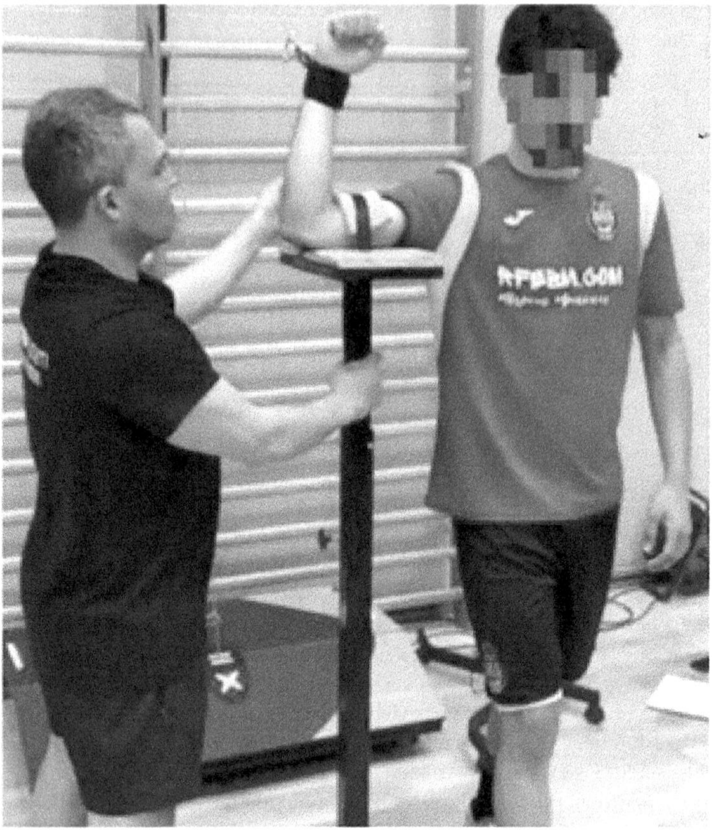

Figure 11.4 Rotator cuff evaluation with FEMD.

Further research, such as the study by García-Buendía et al. (2022), has expanded on these findings by comparing the reliability of different assessment methods. This study explored the influence of shoulder internal rotation strength on throwing velocity, using FEMD to assess the force-velocity profile of the shoulder rotators. Although no direct correlation was found between shoulder strength and throwing velocity, the reliability of the FEMD assessments was confirmed, emphasizing its utility in clinical practice.

The continued validation of FEMD for shoulder assessments not only enhances our diagnostic capabilities but also informs the development of more effective rehabilitation strategies. By integrating such advanced technologies into clinical practice, healthcare providers can achieve better outcomes in the management of shoulder injuries.

References

Andersen, C. H., L. L. Andersen, M. K. Zebis, and G. Sjøgaard. 2014. "Effect of Scapular Function Training on Chronic Pain in the Neck/Shoulder Region: A Randomized Controlled Trial." *Journal of Occupational Rehabilitation* 24 (2): 316–324. doi:10.1007/s10926-013-9441-1.

Bohannon, Richard W., Michal Steffl, Susan S. Glenney, Michelle Green, Leah Cashwell, Kveta Prajerova, and Jennifer Bunn. 2018. "The Prone Bridge Test: Performance, Validity, and Reliability among Older and Younger Adults." *Journal of Bodywork and Movement Therapies* 22 (2). Churchill Livingstone: 385–389. doi:10.1016/j.jbmt.2017.07.005.

Calais-Ferreira, Lucas, Daniel Pozzobon, Marina B. Pinheiro, Fiona M. Blyth, Juan R. Ordoñana, Glen E. Duncan, John L. Hopper, Paulo H. Ferreira, and Manuela L. Ferreira. 2023. "Sex Differences in Lifetime Prevalence of Low Back Pain: A Multinational Study of Opposite-Sex Twin Pairs." *European Journal of Pain* 27 (10). John Wiley & Sons, Ltd: 1150–1160. doi:10.1002/EJP.2146.

Catalá, María Moreno, Arno Schroll, Gunnar Laube, and Adamantios Arampatzis. 2018. "Muscle Strength and Neuromuscular Control in Low-Back Pain: Elite Athletes Versus General Population." *Frontiers in Neuroscience* 12 (JUL). Frontiers Media SA. doi:10.3389/FNINS.2018.00436.

Cho, Kang Hee, Jae Won Beom, Tae Sung Lee, Jun Ho Lim, Tae Heon Lee, and Ji Hyun Yuk. 2014. "Trunk Muscles Strength as a Risk Factor for Nonspecific Low Back Pain: A Pilot Study." *Annals of Rehabilitation Medicine* 38 (2): 234–240. doi:10.5535/arm.2014.38.2.234.

Davies, George J., and Todd S. Ellenbecker. 2012. "Application of Isokinetics in Testing and Rehabilitation." In *Physical Rehabilitation of the Injured Athlete*. Fourth Edition. Elsevier Inc. doi:10.1016/B978-1-4377-2411-0.00025-3.

De Blaiser, Cedric, Roel De Ridder, Tine Willems, Lieven Danneels, and Philip Roosen. 2018. "Reliability and Validity of Trunk Flexor and Trunk Extensor Strength Measurements Using Handheld Dynamometry in a Healthy Athletic Population." *Physical Therapy in Sport* 34 (November). Churchill Livingstone: 180–186. doi:10.1016/j.ptsp.2018.10.005.

Edwards, Anne, Judy Chepeha, Allyson Jones, David M. Sheps, and Lauren Beaupré. 2020. "Can Clinical Assessment Differentiate Partial Thickness Rotator Cuff Tears from Full Thickness Rotator Cuff Tears? A Secondary Analysis." *Disability and Rehabilitation* 42 (16). England: 2351–2358. doi:10.1080/09638288.2018.1563637.

Fehrmann, Elisabeth, Simone Kotulla, Linda Fischer, Thomas Kienbacher, Kerstin Tuechler, Patrick Mair, Gerold Ebenbichler, and Birgit Paul. 2019. "The Impact of Age and Gender on the ICF-Based Assessment of Chronic Low Back Pain." *Disability and Rehabilitation* 41 (10). Taylor & Francis: 1190–1199. doi:10.1080/09638288.2018.1424950.

Ferreira, Manuela L., Katie De Luca, Lydia M. Haile, Jaimie D. Steinmetz, Garland T. Culbreth, Marita Cross, Jacek A. Kopec, et al. 2023. "Global, Regional, and National Burden of Low Back Pain, 1990–2020, Its Attributable Risk Factors, and Projections to 2050: A Systematic Analysis of the Global Burden of Disease Study 2021." *The Lancet Rheumatology* 5 (6): e316–e329. doi:10.1016/S2665-9913(23)00098-X.

García-Buendía, G., D. Martínez-García, D. Jerez-Mayorga, M. Gómez-López, I. J. Chirosa-Ríos, and L. J. Chirosa-Ríos. 2022. "Exploration of the Shoulder Internal Rotation's Influence on Throwing Velocity in Handball Players: A Pilot Study." *International Journal of Environmental Research and Public Health* 19 (23). doi:10.3390/ijerph192315923.

García-Vaquero, María Pilar, David Barbado, Casto Juan-Recio, Alejandro López-Valenciano, and Francisco J. Vera-Garcia. 2020. "Isokinetic Trunk Flexion—Extension Protocol to Assess Trunk Muscle Strength and Endurance: Reliability, Learning Effect, and Sex Differences." *Journal of Sport and Health Science* 9 (6): 692–701. doi:10.1016/j.jshs.2016.08.011.

Hamrick, Mark W., Meghan E. McGee-Lawrence, and Danielle M. Frechette. 2016. "Fatty Infiltration of Skeletal Muscle: Mechanisms and Comparisons with Bone Marrow Adiposity." *Frontiers in Endocrinology* 7 (June). Frontiers Media S.A.: 208170. doi:10.3389/FENDO.2016.00069/BIBTEX.

Hodges, Paul W., and Lieven Danneels. 2019. "Changes in Structure and Function of the Back Muscles in Low Back Pain: Different Time Points, Observations, and Mechanisms." *Journal of Orthopaedic and Sports Physical Therapy* 49 (6). Movement Science Media: 464–476. doi:10.2519/JOSPT.2019.8827/ASSET/IMAGES/LARGE/JOSPT-464-FIG004.JPEG.

Hori, Yusuke, Masatoshi Hoshino, Kazuhide Inage, Masayuki Miyagi, Shinji Takahashi, Shoichiro Ohyama, Akinobu Suzuki, et al. 2019. "ISSLS PRIZE IN CLINICAL SCIENCE 2019: Clinical Importance of Trunk Muscle Mass for Low Back Pain, Spinal Balance, and Quality of Life-a Multicenter Cross-Sectional Study." *European Spine Journal: Official Publication of the European Spine Society, the European Spinal Deformity Society, and the European Section of the Cervical Spine Research Society* 28 (5): 914–921. doi:10.1007/S00586-019-05904-7.

Juan-Recio, Casto, David Barbado Murillo, Alejandro López-Valenciano, and Francisco José Vera-García. 2014. "Test de Campo Para Valorar La Resistencia de Los Músculos Del Tronco." *Apunts Educació Física i Esports*, no. 117 (September). Institut d'Educacio Fisica de Catalunya (INEFC): 59–68. doi:10.5672/APUNTS.2014-0983.ES.(2014/3).117.06.

Juan-Recio, Casto, Diego López-Plaza, David Barbado Murillo, M. Pilar García-Vaquero, and Francisco J. Vera-García. 2017. "Reliability Assessment and Correlation Analysis of 3 Protocols to Measure Trunk Muscle Strength and Endurance." *Journal of Sports Sciences* 36 (4). Routledge: 357–364. doi:10.1080/02640414.2017.1307439.

Kibler, W. Ben, Trevor Wilkes, and Aaron Sciascia. 2013. "Mechanics and Pathomechanics in the Overhead Athlete." *Clinics in Sports Medicine* 32 (4). Elsevier Inc: 637–651. doi:10.1016/j.csm.2013.07.003.

Martinez-Garcia, Dario, Angela Rodriguez-Perea, Paola Barboza, David Ulloa-Díaz, Daniel Jerez-Mayorga, Ignacio Chirosa, and Luis Javier Chirosa Ríos. 2020. "Reliability of a Standing Isokinetic Shoulder Rotators Strength Test Using a Functional Electromechanical Dynamometer: Effects of Velocity." *PeerJ* 8: 1–15. doi:10.7717/peerj.9951.

Mesquita, Marceli M. A., Marta S. Santos, Alan B. S. Vasconcelos, Clodoaldo A. De Sá, Luana C. D. Pereira, Ínea B. M. Da Silva-Santos, Walderi M. Da Silva Junior, et al. 2019. "Reliability of a Test for Assessment of Isometric

Trunk Muscle Strength in Elderly Women." *Journal of Aging Research* 2019. doi:10.1155/2019/9061839.

Owens, Brett D., Scot E. Campbell, and Kenneth L. Cameron. 2013. "Risk Factors for Posterior Shoulder Instability in Young Athletes." *The American Journal of Sports Medicine* 41 (11): 2645–2649. doi:10.1177/0363546513501508.

Reyes-Ferrada, Waleska, L. Chirosa-Rios, I. Chirosa-Rios, D. Martínez-Garcia, Paola Barboza-gonzalez, D. Ulloa-Diaz, Daniel Jerez-mayorga, and A. Rodríguez-Perea. 2022. "A New Reliable Device to Assess Trunk Extensors Strength." *Acta of Bioengineering and Biomechanics* 24 (1): 2022. doi:10.37190/ABB-01965-2021-05.

Reyes-Ferrada, Waleska, Ángela Rodríguez-Perea, Luis Chirosa-Ríos, Darío Martínez-García, and Daniel Jerez-Mayorga. 2022. "Muscle Quality and Functional and Conventional Ratios of Trunk Strength in Young Healthy Subjects: A Pilot Study." *International Journal of Environmental Research and Public Health* 19: 12673. doi:10.3390/ijerph191912673.

Rodríguez-Perea, Angela, María Dolores Morenas Aguilar, Raquel Escobar-Molina, Darío Martínez-García, Ignacio Chirosa Ríos, Daniel Jerez-Mayorga, Luis Chirosa Ríos, Danica Janicijevic, and Waleska Reyes-Ferrada. 2023. "Strength Assessment of Trunk Rotator Muscles: A Multicenter Reliability Study." *Healthcare* 11 (16). Multidisciplinary Digital Publishing Institute: 2331. doi:10.3390/HEALTHCARE11162331.

Rodriguez-Perea, Angela, Luis J. Chirosa Ríos, Dario Martinez-Garcia, David Ulloa-Díaz, Francisco Guede Rojas, Daniel Jerez-Mayorga, and Ignacio J. Chirosa Rios. 2019a. "Reliability of Isometric and Isokinetic Trunk Flexor Strength Using a Functional Electromechanical Dynamometer." *PeerJ* 2019 (10): 1–17. doi:10.7717/peerj.7883.

Roth, Ralf, Lars Donath, Eduard Kurz, Lukas Zahner, and Oliver Faude. 2017. "Absolute and Relative Reliability of Isokinetic and Isometric Trunk Strength Testing Using the IsoMed-2000 Dynamometer." *Physical Therapy in Sport* 24. Elsevier Ltd: 26–31. doi:10.1016/j.ptsp.2016.11.005.

Seitz, Laurent B., and G. Gregory Haff. 2016. "Factors Modulating Post-Activation Potentiation of Jump, Sprint, Throw, and Upper-Body Ballistic Performances: A Systematic Review with Meta-Analysis." *Sports Medicine* 46 (2). Springer International Publishing: 231–240. doi:10.1007/s40279-015-0415-7.

Shaw, Jonathan, Jesse V. Jacobs, Linda R. Van Dillen, George J. Beneck, and Jo Armour Smith. 2023. "Understanding the Biering-Sørensen Test: Contributors to Extensor Endurance in Young Adults with and without Low Back Pain." *MedRxiv*, January. Cold Spring Harbor Laboratory Preprints. doi:10.1101/2023.01.11.23284452.

Steele, James, Stewart Bruce-Low, and Dave Smith. 2014. "A Reappraisal of the Deconditioning Hypothesis in Low Back Pain: Review of Evidence from a Triumvirate of Research Methods on Specific Lumbar Extensor Deconditioning." *Current Medical Research and Opinion* 30 (5): 865–911. doi:10.1185/03007995.2013.875465.

Steeves, Darren, Leo J. Thornley, Joshua A. Goreham, Matthew J. Jordan, Scott C. Landry, and Jonathon R. Fowles. 2019. "Reliability and Validity of a Novel Trunk-Strength Assessment for High-Performance Sprint Flat-Water

Kayakers." *International Journal of Sports Physiology and Performance* 14 (4). Human Kinetics Publishers Inc.: 486–492. doi:10.1123/ijspp.2018-0428.

Verbrugghe, Jonas, Anouk Agten, Bert O. Eijnde, Frank Vandenabeele, Liesbet De Baets, Xavier Huybrechts, and Annick Timmermans. 2019. "Reliability and Agreement of Isometric Functional Trunk and Isolated Lumbar Strength Assessment in Healthy Persons and Persons with Chronic Nonspecific Low Back Pain." *Physical Therapy in Sport* 38 (July). Churchill Livingstone: 1–7. doi:10.1016/J.PTSP.2019.03.009.

Whinton, Alanna K., Kyle M. A. Thompson, Geoffrey A. Power, and Jamie F. Burr. 2018. "Testing a Novel Isokinetic Dynamometer Constructed Using a 1080 Quantum." *PLoS ONE* 13 (7): 1–11. doi:10.1371/journal.pone.0201179.

Zemkova, Erika. 2019. "Reliability of a Novel Method Assessing Muscle Power and Velocity during Seated Trunk Rotations." *Physical Activity Review* 7: 1–8. doi:10.16926/PAR.2019.07.01.

Zemková, Erika, Michal Jelen, Ludmila Zapletalová, and Dusan Hamar. 2017. "Muscle Power during Standing and Seated Trunk Rotations with Different Weights." *Sport Mont* 15 (3): 17–23. doi:10.26773/smj.2017.10.003.

Zhu, Wan-Ping, Yue Huang, Peng Hu, and Wei Lin. 2023. "Lumbar Extensor and Flexor Muscle Structural Changes in Young Female Nurses with Chronic Bilateral Non-Specific Low Back Pain: A Case-Control Study." *Discovery Medicine* 35 (176): 444–450. doi:10.24976/Discov.Med.202335176.45.

Index

Note: Page numbers in *italics* indicate a figure and page numbers in **bold** indicate a table on the corresponding page.

For Product Safety Concerns and Information please contact our EU representative GPSR@taylorandfrancis.com
Taylor & Francis Verlag GmbH, Kaufingerstraße 24, 80331 München, Germany

www.ingramcontent.com/pod-product-compliance
Lightning Source LLC
LaVergne TN
LVHW021127300926
849160LV00010B/892